Ties
That
Bind

Ties
That
Bind

The SM/Leather/Fetish Erotic Style

Issues, Commentaries and Advice

Guy Baldwin, M.S.

Edited by Joseph Bean

Preface by Gayle Rubin

Daedalus Publishing Company
2140 Hyperion Ave.
Los Angeles, CA 90027

Published by Daedalus Publishing Company, 2140 Hyperion Ave. Los Angeles, CA 90027

Cover design by Don Mooring

ISBN 1-881943-09-7

Library of Congress Catalog Card Number: 93-70930

Printed in the United States of America

These efforts are dedicated to Jim Kane and Ike Barns, my first mentors—still together after 21 years—and to all my departed brethren. I could hardly list or properly memorialize them all here, but I offer as a dedication *in memoriam* a note I wrote for *Drummer* on the passing of Jim Ed Thompson.

In the summer of '77, I set up a scene between Jim Ed and my then lover as my birthday present to my main man. Jim Ed met him at a bar, put an eyeless hood on my lover, drove him around a while, then drove him to my house. Jim threw him over one shoulder and carried him into my playroom for a hot scene. My lover had no idea where he was, and I got to watch Jim play with him for several hours. Later, Jim and I ate birthday pie off my lover's chest with great relish—candles burning all the while. I shall never forget...never.

Today, I learned of Jim Ed's death, and a part of me went with him, for he has been one of the village elders, a keeper of the sacred flame. I took my Harley up through Griffith Park earlier on a sort of memorial ride. I listened to the wind whistling past my ears—listened for any whispering that may have been there, rather like the oracles at Delphi, leaning over that crack in the earth, inhaling the vapors, hopeful of some sign. I heard sounds, but I do not know what they meant.

I tried to think on what might make my sorrow lighter, and suddenly I thought of Jim Ed playing with my friends Larry Hunt, Bruce Rapp, Mike Cahalin, and other village elders who have also left. And, lo, a smile graced my sad, wet lips.

I shall do Thirteen Strokes, and smartly, in your honor this year at Inferno. Good-bye, my Friend.

Guy Baldwin

ACKNOWLEDGEMENTS

To write anything of consequence, one must have help and support from others. For me, these must include my leather family, friends, colleagues, lovers, suitors, Tops, bottoms, Masters, slaves, and some special acquaintances.

Specifically, they are: Scot Answer, Mikal Bales, Race Bannon, Ike Barnes, Joseph Bean, Bear, Mike Boustead, David Britton D.M.A., Jim Burnett M.D., Jeff Burnham, Roger Burroughs, john burrow, Pat Califia, Steve Darrow, Brian Dawson, Durk Dehner, Barry Douglas, George Fouras M.D., Vince Gaither, Chris Hanson, Marcus Hernandez, Larry Hunt, Andrew Irish, Ron Johnson, Jim Kane, Fred Katz, Don Levi, Wes Lockwood, Jan Lyon, Tom Magister, Dwayne McWaine M.D., Mike Pereyra, Mike Pierce, Matoc Pope, Mariano Rabino, Chuck Renslow, Henry Romanowski, Gayle Rubin, Will Russell, Dorothy Satten Ph.D., Tony Scarcella M.D., Bobby Smith—The Elder, Bob Smith—The Younger, Robert Stoller M.D., Jim-Ed Thompson, Mark Thompson, Jim Ward, and David Willoughby. Some of these are already gone but not forgotten.

Thanks and deep appreciation must also go to my clients who teach me constantly; members of the Chicago Hellfire Club, and those who have been kind enough to find my work suitable for publication. Thank you all.

Pictures From The Black Dance

I am the painter; come now, my canvas.
Trophied whiteness, to sweat in zenith Sun.
You are my medium, treasured seer
From the workshop of your mother's womb.

Destined to my hand this hour
To caress; to play; to coax
Sweet throat's surrender song;
Your Magic Lyric, to free us both.

Expert eyes scan sacred tools, judging
Which will loose your writhing lust,
Transcend tormented craving, and
By agonized flight be blessed.

Your favored cat finds my hand.
Eyes meet; a signal passes;
Entre, adagio, variation, coda.
Guts 'cross dorsal sinews land.

Swirling Delphic ethers rise;
Sonic picture. Listen, eyes!
Miss nothing. No twitch slips by,
No sound unseen. A catch; a cry.

Comes now a vision, crimson map.
Ascent begins; scream thunderclap.
Travelers two, enchantment found;
To rapture's portal again we're bound.

TABLE OF CONTENTS

Pictures from the Black Dance

Preface by Gayle Rubin   15

The Editor's Introduction to *Ties That Bind*   19

Author's Note   23

Part One: The Relationship Essays

Editor's Note on The Relationship Essays   27

A Second Coming Out   31
From *Frontiers*, September, 1989, and *Leatherfolk*, 1991

Let's Get Real   41
From *Drummer* #110, *Ties That Bind*, dated 10/87

Outside, Looking In?   47
From *Drummer* #127, *Ties That Bind*, dated 04/89

Let's Not Take the Olde Guard Judges Too Seriously   51
From *Drummer* #112, *Ties That Bind*, dated 01/88

Blindman's Bluff Hurts Too Much   55
From *Drummer* #111, *Ties That Bind*, dated 12/87

Men Who Switch: Treasures and Tribulations   59
From *Drummer* #117, *Ties That Bind*, dated 06/88

Three Or More?   65
From *Drummer* #152, *Ties That Bind*, dated 02/92

Master/slave Relationships: An Overview   71
From *Drummer* #118, *Ties That Bind*, dated 07/88

Master/slave Relationships: Warnings   77
From *Drummer* #119, *Ties That Bind*, dated 07/88

When Partners Play Together   85
From *Drummer* #116, *Ties That Bind*, dated 05/88

Smoothing Out the Rough Spots   91
From *Drummer* #151, *Ties That Bind*, dated 10/91

Part Two: The Community Commentaries

Editor's Note on The Community Commentaries   99

Glass Houses   101
From *Drummer* #135, *Ties That Bind*, dated 12/89

"Old Guard": Its Origins, Traditions, Mystique & Rules   107
From *Drummer* #150, *Rear View Mirror*, dated 09/91

Teach Them a Little Bit   117
From *Drummer* #128, *Ties That Bind*, dated 05/89

A Leather Family?   123
From *Drummer* #132, *Ties That Bind*, dated 08/89

SM and Child Abuse   127
From *Drummer* #154, *Sane Sex*, dated 04/92

Beauties & Beasts Revisited   131
From *Manifest Reader* #10

Leather In the '90s: Another View   137
For *Manifest Reader* (unpublished)

Political Scat: Or Is There Really Anything But   143
the Smell?
From *The Leather Journal* #41, dated 12/92

Part Three: On Enhancing The SM Experience

Editor's Note on On Enhancing The SM Experience   151

You Go Together, Or You Don't Go At All!   153
Composed of *Ties That Bind* from *Drummer* #121-123,
Fall 1988

Who's Running This Show, Anyway?   167
From *Drummer* #126, *Ties That Bind*, dated 03/89

Tops: Out In the Cold?   171
From *Drummer* #124 *Ties That Bind*, dated 12/88

The Trouble With Tops   175
From *Drummer* #115, *Ties That Bind*, dated 04/88

Beware the Killer Bottom   181
From *Drummer* #113, *Ties That Bind*, dated 02/88

Thinking About Consent   185
From *Drummer* #131, *Ties That Bind*, dated 07/89

Pushing Limits: When Consent Can Get In the Way   191
From *Checkmate* #3, dated 04/93

Some Straight Talk About Drugs   197
From *Drummer* #125, *Ties That Bind*, dated 02/89

The Mental Side Of Playing "Safe" & "Sane"   203
From *Drummer* #153, Feature Article, dated 03/92

Humiliation: What's In It For You?   209
From *Drummer* #114, *Ties That Bind*, dated 03/88

Punishment: Proceed With Caution!   213
From *Drummer* #120, *Ties That Bind*, dated 08/88

Part Four: Catapulting Toward Transformation

Editor's Note on Catapulting Toward Transformation   221

To Ecstasy And Beyond: One Road Map   223
From *Checkmate* #2, dated 02/93

Fear Is the Enemy   229
From *Drummer* #155, *Rough Stuff*, dated 05/92

In My Father's House, There Are Many Mansions   237
From *Drummer* #136, *Ties That Bind*, dated 01/90

About the Author   241

PREFACE

"The future lies in kinky people."

—*Personal Services* 1986 (National Film
Trustee Company)

Many people think of Guy Baldwin as a major leather titleholder in the late 1980's. But while the title system confers moments of high (if fleeting) visibility, Guy has a much longer, more varied, and more interesting leather career.

I first met Guy in San Francisco in 1978, through networks that crossed and mingled by way of the Society of Janus. I remember him as a slender man in impeccable leathers, cap drawn low over dark sunglasses, a Presence with a penetrating gaze and an impenetrable attitude. In addition to his involvement in the mixed gender/mixed orientation Society of Janus, Guy had by then already spent many years in the world of gay male leather. After he entered that community in the mid-sixties, he had the good fortune to be schooled and taught by some of the finest exemplars of old guard gay male leather.

I would occasionally run into Guy after he moved to Los Angeles in 1980. But I began to know him better in the heady days of the early National Leather Association (NLA) gatherings. In 1987, we were both attending the second NLA Living in Leather (LIL) conference. I was astonished to find that he had become a hunky, muscular, bodybuilder. He had also become a practicing psychotherapist in Los Angeles, where his clients were mostly other kinky gay men.

Guy subsequently became a regular columnist for *Drummer* magazine, Mr. National Leather Association 1989-90, and International Mr. Leather 1989. Throughout all his many changes, Guy has remained very much as I first remembered him: an immensely passionate, powerful, thoughtful, and articulate personality who has committed much of his life and

15

work to the advancement of kinky people.

During seminars and workshops for leather organizations and at conferences, Guy began actively to share some of the insights gleaned from his experience and from his therapy practice. He also began to write a series of remarkable articles in *Drummer* magazine. His column, "Ties that Bind," was one of the most compelling features of *Drummer* in the late eighties and early nineties. Just as I had rushed, a decade earlier, to read the latest installment of *Mr. Benson*, I greedily examined each new issue of *Drummer* for Guy's latest musings on the leather condition. He kept addressing many issues with which I and my friends wrestled, but which were infrequently brought up in public leather or SM forums.

Guy's writing is an important contribution to a maturing self awareness among leatherfolk of all genders and orientations. The earliest leather oriented literature was erotic, and was fashioned to elicit sexual excitement. While literature and art dedicated solely to sexual pleasure are to be treasured, they are not usually designed to meet other needs. By the late seventies, an elaborate technical literature arrived as a welcome addition to the older tradition of person-to-person transmission of information about how to do SM, bondage, and fetish play.

Most other commentary was polemical, and was aimed at creating and disseminating moral and political justifications for leather, SM, and fetish predilections. This was important, not only to mitigate the general social hostility toward kinky folk, but also to help practitioners feel better about being kinky and doing kinky things. As Guy has said, "the freedom to be different and feel OK about it must be fought for."

Nevertheless, at times the leather, SM, and fetish communities become mesmerized by their own rhetoric. Stigmatized populations often begin their march toward acceptance by agitating to replace negative stereotypes with positive ones. But the gay movement had to move beyond simple affirmations such as "gay is good" to more nuanced understandings of the joys and sorrows and variety of gay and lesbian life. Similarly, the leather/SM/fetish movement needs the luxury of deeper and more complex discussions of the unique pleasures, particular pitfalls, and endless diversity of what we call, for lack of a better term, "leather." This collection of Guy Baldwin's meditations is indicative of a growing inclination in the leather villages to grapple with a broader range of experiences, problems, and possibilities, some of which are difficult to identify, describe and explain.

Although Guy's personal history and professional work are predominantly among gay men, his gutsy honesty and intelligence make his observations relevant to kinky people of all persuasions. It is not only gay leathermen who struggle with issues such as how to enter into scenes, how to set and recognize limits, the emotional needs of Tops and bottoms, the dangers of "SM correctness," bottom problems and problem bottoms, Top problems and problem Tops, SM relationships, multiple partners, switching, the subtleties of consent, emotional safety, SM and personal histories of childhood abuse, SM and mental/emotional health, the distinctions between fantasies and behaviors, and the imperative role of honest self knowledge and direct communication for satisfying SM play.

Issues of sexual, stylistic, and community diversity have become more salient as the different kinky populations increasingly encounter one another in social, political, and sexual contexts. Generational change and succession must be confronted by all human groups, but it has idiosyncratic manifestations among people for whom certain icons of the 1950's have been such potent fulcrums of sexual desire and community formation.

Guy is at his best when he explores arcana of the dynamics of SM/fetish/bondage scenes. Many serious players contemplate the sometimes fine distinctions between SM and abuse, or wonder how to communicate when limits shift, or ponder the dynamic tensions between the boundaries of agreement and the portals of rapture. Experienced players often seek those elusive, transcendent, and ecstatic experiences which can occur when sexual energy goes into overdrive. Guy offers practical emotional and technical suggestions for navigating these perilous outer banks, and for returning safely. There is plenty of wise advice in this book for both veterans and beginners. Kinky women, men, and transgendered people who are gay, lesbian, bisexual, heterosexual, polymorphous, or indeterminate will all find much to savor here.

Guy is a rare fellow. His roots are in the most venerable strata of the leather world; yet he is fully engaged with the issues of the present. He speaks in a contemporary voice, with a strong sense of the past and with a rare eloquence. I do not always agree with Guy; but I never fail to learn from him.

Gayle Rubin
San Francisco 1993

The Editor's Introduction to
Ties That Bind

There are questions an editor—or any reader, for that matter—must ask when faced with a new book: Why was this book written? Why should it be published? What does it have to offer readers which they cannot already find elsewhere? From the editor's point of view, the answers to these questions are vital. They give him something to work toward as he makes the hundreds of decisions and choices that give the text its final form.

The best reason for any book being written is that there are readers in need of the information it will include, in search of that information in the author's voice, or—regardless of whether they see a need or mount a search—readers who will significantly benefit from the book if they are exposed to it.

There are many people who need what Guy Baldwin presents here. They know they need it because they have already undertaken leather/SM lifestyles, and need some guidance. They want to do SM, to be able to invoke the pleasures and the gods, to stir the spirits and the energies, without too great a risk of also summoning the destruction that seems always to gather in the shadows of a scene, waiting for anything like an invitation.

There are also many people actively searching for Baldwin's voice and perspective—the tone that comes from his loving-kindness, the edge that comes with his intense experience in the scene, and the insight that comes from his training and work as a psychotherapist. I know the searchers are out there because I have heard from them. During my years as editor of *Drummer*, and in the years before, I encountered a great many people who wanted to know what mental health professionals thought of SM. As the number of Baldwin's articles published in *Drummer* grew, so did the requests for specifically those back issues in which his "Ties that Bind" column had appeared.

As for the third category of possible benefactors of this book, those who may not know enough to hunger for the information or suspect its existence, they too are many. As SM and the leather subculture become increasingly visible by way of television shows like *LA Law* and *Law and Order*, through the success of books like Madonna's *Sex*, and in ads, popular music, dance clubs, and the like, more and more people are giving radical sex a whirl. For the most part, they don't start out aware of any need to be educated, but the more they know the better. If they can be induced to read books like this one, there will be far fewer unintentional scars, and fewer psychological accidents.

I sincerely hope that I have introduced no errors to this text in my effort to make it accessible to the widest possible readership. I further hope that I have not strained or unduly altered Baldwin's beautifully warped, not to say eccentric, way with the English language. Some conventions—like the big-T for the word Top as contrasted with the little-b for bottom, and the fact that the language is usually cast in a male-primary form—might easily be misunderstood. Since all of the essays here were written by a gay, male leatherman, almost all of them for a gay, male, leather-inclined readership, certain conventions and stylistic choices were entirely appropriate. Much of what was appropriate to the original publication of the essays has become integral to their style.

No anti-female or anti-feminist leanings on the part of the author, editor, or publisher should be inferred. Women, male and female heterosexuals and bisexuals, and transgenderal folks; young people, older people, and those new to leather/SM; Old Guard gay leathermen, and the most radical of New Leather seekers will all find the material here valuable. Indeed, if it were satisfactory for this material to be offered only to gay men already settled in the leather lifestyles, there would be little need for this book. On the other hand, any attempt to stretch the language to refer *in all cases* to all possible readers, would weaken or destroy the sense of the text, or at least impede immediate understanding. I have chosen wherever the question arose to err on the side of retaining the original language rather than risk the unforgivable error of obfuscation. After all, what matters here is the communication of ideas, not the sex or orientation of the thinker or his audience.

Finally, I am deeply grateful to Guy Baldwin and Race Bannon for trusting me with this manuscript, and to my slave warren for keeping the editorial process on track when we might both have liked to be doing other things. I have enjoyed working on *Ties That Bind*, and—even though I had already read all but three of the pieces in this book—I have learned a good deal about myself and my sexuality by becoming intimate with Baldwin on the computer screen and on the printed page.

Joseph W. Bean
February 3, 1993
San Francisco

Author's Note

For those who have a mission in life, sometimes the burden of that mission is light, and sometimes not. My mission has been to illuminate, as best I can, the path toward self-awareness via responsible and thoughtful explorations of the SM/fetish erotic style. Like most people with a mission, I discovered that I had been traveling that path a while before I came to realize the exact nature and scope of the mission itself.

It began with a small circle of close friends who were interested in my opinions about the SM experience; then it grew to include their acquaintances. The clinic where I completed my internship invited me to offer a series of drop-in discussion groups on leathersex-related topics, here for the first time, I began to share my ideas with strangers. Soon, I found that I was receiving requests to address a local SM organization.

The circle of acquaintances grew to include the publisher of *Drummer* magazine who asked me to write a column, and I agreed. Suddenly I found that I had become separated from my audience by time and space; they had become "readers." I had gone from sharing intimate opinions with a small circle of friends to casting out messages in a paper bottle in the span of 16 years. It was partly this growing feeling of isolation that called me to become International Mr. Leather in 1989; thus, I re-established an all-important contact with the members of my tribe.

About three years after my column began appearing in *Drummer*, people everywhere started asking me if there were plans to publish them as a collection some day. This question always surprised me, and I always answered in the negative. I found it hard to believe that the articles were that important. After all, I was just telling the truth as I had come to understand it. But finally, the pressure to publish these and some other writing in a collection was too great to ignore; here it is at last. And so, the circle grows again.

However it has come about, it is my most sincere hope that

at least some of the ideas contained in the following material will be of use to you in your own journey toward yourself. This was, after all, the point of the writing in the first place.

Although most of my work collected in this book was originally written with the gay leatherman in mind, I know that many others with different erotic identities will find things of value. Please translate the pronouns as necessary.

Guy Baldwin, M.S.
Los Angeles 1993

Part One

THE RELATIONSHIP ESSAYS

Editor's Note On
The Relationship Essays

Guy began writing for *Drummer* because Anthony F. DeBlase, then both publisher and editor of the magazine, wanted him to write a column about SM relationships. Baldwin's credentials were impeccable. He was—and is—a very much respected psychotherapist, often working with people whose problems involve SM play and/or relationships which either do (and that's the problem) or don't (and that's the problem) accommodate SM well.

It is unclear whether his writing for *Drummer* led to his writing for *Frontiers, The Leather Journal, Checkmate*, or any other publications. What is clear is that his column in *Drummer* led a great many readers to re-examine themselves and their relationships, to look more frankly and honestly at what was real and what was not even desirable—however much it might look delicious in fantasy. And, obviously, not every reader became a fan. Some people would rather dream, however uncomfortably, than face life as it is.

In any case, he wrote, always with authority, sometimes with great power, often about things that left people feeling powerless until they were given the keys to understanding. In the course of the writing, he coined many phrases and was forced to strain ordinary language to accommodate the subjects and interests he was trying to address. (He also popularized the non-purjorative use of the word kinky in his writing and his lectures, by the way.) Many words have been left as written, and outsiders to the SM scene may find some at least unusual. For the most part, these words are left to be defined by the context in which they are used. A few, however, deserve to be mentioned here, before you encounter them in the text.

Top and *bottom* as they refer to sexual partners, for instance, are words easily enough understood by most people. Still, those who are not familiar with the traditions of the leather community may get a wrong impression when they see that Top (the active partner in the usual sense of the word) is always capitalized, and bottom (the passive partner) is always begun with a lower case letter. This is not an implication that bottoms are less than Tops, less valuable, less human, less important, or whatever. It is merely a convention with which leathermen express the dominant/submissive characters implied by the words. Capital-T Tops preside over lower-case-b bottoms, but only by the consent and willing participation of the bottoms. Don't be offended; try to catch the spirit intended instead.

Another word some readers may find offensive is *vanilla*. No offense is intended. Just as gay people settled on (and, more recently have begun to reject) *straight* as a word to refer to those who are not gay, leatherfolk are (for now) settled on vanilla as the descriptive for those who are not kinky (involved in radical sex). It is just a word for lack of any better one, and the whole leather community is listening for any genuine improvement on the term.

Finally, a word that is used in leather circles a great deal is *scene*. The confusion caused by this word is endless when leatherfolk are talking to vanilla people, but minimal in leather-to-leather conversations. The scene can refer to the whole leather/SM/fetish/radical sex world, as when a person asks "is he/she *in the scene?*" Or it can refer to a single experience of leathersex, an encounter, as when a leatherman says "the scene with him was really intense." Only context will separate the two meanings of the word, but knowing both definitions exist is all that you will require for understanding.

As to the letters S and M, the problem is not so difficult when the writer is Guy Baldwin. SM generally means sadomasochism. Some people would say it ought to mean Sex Magic. Others will claim that it properly means Sensuality/Mutuality. The truth is that, with this writer, you are safe to include all you own meanings in the letter S and M (knowing that he is aware of and inclusive of them too), except where he is very specific about a narrower definition.

It has been my intention as the editor of the essays in this section, and the remainder of the book, to leave the text as much in its original, published form as is consistent with the basic needs of the general reader. I have been encouraged to change everything to make it easily accessible to all, and equally encouraged to change nothing to retain the sense and mentality of the original. I have chosen to steer a near-middle course, leaving Guy Baldwin's thoughts to reach out, and encourage you to think with him about—in this section—SM relationships.

A Second Coming Out

I remember quite well the progression of events by which I came into this world—the world of Leatherdomain. In a way, it began with the whispered cautions intended to warn me away from what would (reportedly) result in the wreckage of my life. I was 18 at the time and lived in Denver.

These warnings from my sweater bar acquaintances about "leather queens" were uttered with what I thought was an odd mixture of tittering scorn, awe and suspicion. Leather types, they said, were to be avoided. Even if no one seemed to know quite why, they meant trouble. My bar friends would just roll their eyes heavenward when pressed for details.

The warnings frightened, but also tantalized me. I had secret desires—desires that I knew my friends did not share. These longings were not yet specific, but they held my erotic attention the way gravity holds the Earth in its orbit: strongly, silently, invisibly. I felt gripped by something at once both scary and exciting.

I know that lesbians and gay men alike will understand this because the feelings are the same as when we are just coming out into gay life for the first time. In fact, for those who are already gay or lesbian, the act of acknowledging our kinkiness is a second coming out, which is accompanied by all the same sorts of fear, stress, excitement, and hiding.

Then I had my first adult kinky encounter with myself. After awakening one morning in a trick's apartment, I wandered into his bathroom and was quite surprised to catch sight in his mirror of some rather significant finger nail scratches on my back that I must have gotten sometime during the sex. I couldn't look *at* them, and I couldn't look away. Once I knew they were there, I could actually feel them with my mind. I left his apartment hurriedly, fearing that he would find my fascination sick.

I raced home. There, I twisted myself into various positions to see the marks in my own small mirror, and to touch the scratches where I could reach. Their tingling was distantly familiar. I remembered the childhood wiggling of a loose tooth, just on the edge of pain, yet dreamily pleasurable. As I recalled this, I also remembered that I would tease such a tooth many times during a day. It hurt so good. And thus, my journey began with those few virginal scratches.

After that first wiggly tooth
Finally does fall out,
We await the next one
With anxious anticipation.
I will never believe
I was excited about the Tooth Fairy.
For me, I know it was the wiggle.

The trophy-scratches from that definitive encounter faded into my past as they healed during the next several days. I felt a loss. This single experience began to clarify the vague longings I had felt for years but which had always been without name or focus.

But the scratches had been incidental to our shared moments of passion—accidental and unintended. I began to wonder if the hurt-so-good experience could be controlled, managed, refined. Could such energies be harnessed? I don't know how, but I felt certain that those "leather types" I had been warned about knew something about the mixture of passion and sex with pain, pleasure and sensuality. I sensed that I was standing on the shores of a Sea of Sensuality. I wished to swim but not to drown. Then, I remembered the warnings, and I got scared. But there was no need. I was safer than I realized.

Urban Knights

My introduction to leather life was really my introduction

32

to leather *bar* life. Twenty five years ago, they were one and the same. Now, fortunately, they are not.

A leather bar is not usually an easy place to walk into for the first time, especially when you sense that you are in search of some part of yourself—as I was. Many of the guys look tough and threatening although very, very few are even slightly dangerous.

Then, as now, I was surprised and delighted to discover conversation in leather bars that ranged from carburetors to *Carmen*, from *Mary Poppins* to Mary, Queen of Scots, and from particle board to particle accelerators.

Perhaps it was my own over-active romantic imagination, but those guys seemed like Renaissance men cast as urban knights astride their iron horses. Those who weren't college smart were street smart. It was a good mix. Taken as a group, they supplied all that had been missing in my own family: the capacity for honesty with little or no pretense; spontaneity; and, often enough, a fearless interest in the world and its possibilities.

The motorcycles and leather gear certainly did get my attention. But it was riveted by the heady sex energy that drifted through the hangouts like the sweet smell of boy sweat in a locker room at school. Only these were grown up boys—really men. And always, the black leather, organic armor. It is no accident that the men and women of many religious orders wear black—often a holy color, it seems.

The chance of being accepted as a man among these particular men became more electrifying when I realized that there were some unspoken rites of passage to be experienced that involved sex, and something more. I didn't know just what "more" meant, but I was anxious to find out. I hoped that I would be allowed to learn. Eventually I was.

I came to learn that an SM encounter is my chance to have an intense physical and psychological experience that is mixed with primal sex energy. These energies, often combined with ritual, can be harnessed to produce feelings including the achievement of ecstacy, bonding, altered states of consciousness, and deep meditation. A "scene" (a kinky encounter) is often hypnotic and may have a therapeutic effect in the lives of the players—it certainly has in mine. It seems to me that when they work well, leather and SM sexualities are about transformation. Only recently have some of us begun to acknowledge and discuss this feature of these sexualities among ourselves.

It is little wonder that we sometimes refer to them as religious experiences, because that's what they feel like. Those who are transformed by the rites of passage that I went searching for over 20 years ago have come to form a kind of fraternity—a brotherhood or sisterhood of those who have traveled within to confront the Inner Self.

New Age Leather

By the late '60s, some leathermen began having spiritual experiences and some spiritual guys began to have leather and SM experiences. Through this happy development, a number of us realized that the leather and SM scene could serve us as a meditation path.

When leather and SM scenes were done in a certain way, we achieved a different level of awareness—we felt transformed into someone whom it felt better to be. Also, a kind of bonding occurred between SM players that had been missing in our more usual sexual encounters.

Some of us referred to it as "the SM High" because when it happened, it felt similar to, but better than the best drug experiences we had shared earlier with LSD (acid) and other psychedelic drugs during the '60s. Because the element of ecstatic transformation was common to these experiences, they felt spiritual to many of us. The "religious" leather and SM experience was born.

Our critics have often sneered at the suggestion that leather, SM, and/or fetish sexuality can be the basis of greater spiritual awareness. Such sneering is merely kink-o-phobia, a fear of erotic variation. Yet, anthropologists have long told us about religious ecstasy being achieved by means of physical and mental stress. Transformation through ritual ordeal is an established fact dating back to before the development of writing.

It is very much alive in modern religious practice today. Men from Italy to Japan vie for the honor of sharing in the struggle as they carry heavy religious symbols through neighborhood streets during special sacred ceremonies. Some Catholics and Hindus walk great distances on bloodied knees over sacred pilgrimage routes as an act of penance, for purification, or merely as a sign of devotion—many arrive at holy places in a religious ecstasy. Monks and nuns from numerous religious orders routinely scourge themselves for spiritual purposes. Hindu religious festivals sometimes include men covered with flesh-piercing spikes which support a heavy headdress. Some Native American sacred ceremonies call for physically punishing ceremonies ranging from the flesh-tearing Sun Dance ceremony to the ritual whipping of the Kachina. Until rather recently, fasting was part of every Catholic's religious experience. The anthropological record is replete with examples of this same phenomenon, ritual ordeal coupled with spiritual transformation, even among culturally isolated groups. Certainly, at least some SM explorations compare with practices of the Tantrics and the Shivaites, and connect with the role of chastity in religious life, the rites of Dionysus and rituals of other pagan religions. (Remember, "pagan" merely means not Christian, Jewish or Muslim.)

It is not surprising that many people with a fervent Christian background end up at least sniffing around the leather and SM scene. After all, many Christian sects urge their followers to be like Christ, and they all learn about His passion and suffering. Ever wondered how a crown of thorns might feel, or had fantasies about crucifixion?

For what it's worth, I am acquainted with five members of the Christian clergy—three of them Catholic priests—who are very much into the leather and SM scene. From what I have been able to observe, these men suffer no apparent spiritual conflict, and are altogether fine guys who are bright, interesting, have a good sense of humor, and seem as psychologically well-adjusted as anyone else.

What do new age leathermen do in the search for these ecstatic and transforming scenes? What do we seek? For well over a decade, some of us have been learning how to harness the hurts-so-good feeling through the refinement and control of both physical and mental stress usually in an erotic, ritual setting or context. More specifically, bondage and SM techniques are used to stress the body and (or) dominance and submission are used to stress the mind. When done correctly, the ecstatic transformation occurs.

Despite the AIDS crisis, valuable progress has been made in the search for information about the connection between spiritual awareness and leather, SM and fetish sexualities. When the spiritual aspects of these sexualities are given attention, they can add to who we are as people by increasing our capacity for intimacy and in many other ways. Sexualities that keep us apart only diminish us as people.

It has been suggested that those of us who pursue ecstatic spiritual or mystical experience through leather, SM or fetish activities may be the early forerunners of a new spiritual tradition. It is more likely that at first accidentally, now more purposively, we combine many pre-existing elements in perhaps a new way and give it all an erotic spin to make it work. For now, we are still too close to it to understand it absolutely. Like all early explorers, we do not know what lays ahead, but we know that the path is somehow correct.

A Community Comes of Age

In the '50s and '60s, things were very different from now. There were no overt leather or SM publications, no leather or SM organizations, no politics, no discussion groups, no how-to videos, no poetry, and only a few photocopied porno stories that were passed around.

The leather icons of Tom of Finland and Luger were just

36

beginning to appear in out of the way places in the early '70s. [Editor's note: While Tom of Finland drawings actually first appeared in the US in the late 1950s, they were little known in leather circles at the time. Luger, a more explicitly* leather-oriented artist arrived on the scene much later.] It was a fledgling subculture, confined mostly to the 10 or 12 leather bars around the country.

Today, the leather liberation movement is approximately where the mainstream gay and lesbian community was two decades ago. Although leatherfolk have not had a "Stonewall" as such, we are indisputably becoming tribal. The men's bike club scene was certainly where this community building process began in the late '40s. Gay bikers in leather banded together in nationwide networks, and you may be certain that some of those guys were kinky. These days, it isn't just leather and motorcycles; now, rubber, cowboy gear, tatoos, piercings and even spandex to some extent have become the tribal markings for those with these leather and/or SM sensibilities.

All this change, this maturation, is happening for the same reasons that movement happened among mainstream gays and lesbians in the '60s. People with similar interests are talking with each other about what really matters to them—a healthy process from my point of view. And, while our sexualities are still listed as psychological disturbances in the official reference texts, there has been some progress made there, too. Let us not forget that homosexuality was considered an illness until quite recently.

Like lesbians and gay men, we kinky people are seen by most of the world as sick and dangerous in various (usually unspecified) ways. That is why we are shunned, feared, and hated. When we agree with outsiders that we are sick we soon come to shun, fear and hate ourselves, too. It's called "gay homophobia" when gays hate gayness. For us, I'll call it kink-o-phobia when we hate our own erotic differentness. Self-hate in anyone's life produces the predictable result of serious ego damage.

The real question in the discussion about what is and is not sick is this: For whom is the behavior a problem?. If, for example, a buddy and I look forward to a Saturday night of play with our favorite boots, boot polish, rags, and lube, and have no unsafe sex, then who is to criticize? It might not be your cup of tea, but so what? It must be for us to decide. Until there is *responsible* erotic self-determination for all adults, it will not really exist for anyone.

I emphatically do not mean to suggest that all kinky people are the picture of psychological health. To do so would be equivalent to suggesting that there is no mental illness among gay people; all professional clinicians know better. Just as there are many unhealthy ways for gays to behave with gayness, so too are there many unhealthy ways for kinky people to behave with sexual encounters of the kinky kind.

Subcultures always develop their own morality as has happened in the lesbian and gay communities. The kinky tribes have done so, too. The national leather and SM movement has somehow agreed on three general principals that we use to guide our explorations of these sexualities. They are: safe, sane, and consensual.

Loosely, safe means that sufficient care is taken to prevent accidental or unwanted physical or psychological injury and that procedures be followed that prevent the transmission of disease. Sane means that those who play together are mentally in charge of themselves; that they are also not under the influence of any substances to excess. Consensual, means that any player has the ability to influence the pace, intensity and direction of an erotic encounter at all times, and may end it at will, or say "No" in the first place. Modern day players exploring the sexual frontier would do well to avoid anyone who does not or will not subscribe to these ideals in advance.

It has been the new-age leather folks who have developed a code of morality, self-restraint, and inclusion through the principals of safe, sane and consensual action. The new agers have been influential in the creation and management of many leather and SM organizations, and this has encouraged communication, diversity, and variety to bloom. A new consciousness is moving through the leather scene and is slowly changing the way that leather folks relate to each other both in and out of the playroom.

Ending the Silence

People are most likely to have trouble in the kinky world when they operate as loners and do not make friends within the community, or when there is a lack of emotional maturity. Secret lives make for secret suffering, and the time for secrets about who we are and what we enjoy is slowly ending. Kinky folks (gays more than non-gays) have begun to follow mainstream lesbians and gays out of the closet. If living a lie is bad for anyone, then it must be bad for everyone. But first, we must come out to ourselves, to claim the truth of our erotic reality. This is the implicit message of Stonewall, and leather and SM people are learning the lesson well. This process began in the '70s and continued all through the '80s.

Consequently, we now have conferences, fund raisers, swap meets, workshops, fly-in play parties, and technical demonstrations. There are mail order suppliers, seminars, specialty contact publications, erotic art, and sub-culture heros. We have writers, physicians, lawyers, therapists, toy makers, poets and songwriters, philosophers, and liturgists too. And, of course, we are well into the refinement of our various sexualities.

There are several how-to publications and over 200 clubs and organizations in the U.S. and at least half that number abroad. At last, there are numerous sources of information and guidance that help explorers avoid the problems that can sometimes make the kinky world a singularly unrewarding ordeal.

Clearly, one of the most significant changes to happen is that some kinky gay men and lesbians are finally talking to (and, more rarely, playing next to) each other. Some of us are beginning to discover that common interests in our erotic variation are sometimes more important than whether we are

39

men or women. Kinky heterosexual folks have discovered that they have much to learn from their lesbian and gay male counterparts. And all of us are teaching each other in a number of cautiously experimental settings.

What most non-kinky people don't know is that exploration of leather and SM erotic themes can function in the same self-revealing way that any other sexuality works. It is no accident that among practitioners of this sex style, we may often describe SM as meaning "Sensuality and Mutuality" or "Sexual Magic." More and more, kinky people who enjoy these sexualities feel that they add to who we are as people, not subtract. The absence of guilt and fear is making a big difference. Sound familiar?

No one will ever know how much suffering has been eliminated through the efforts of what we once called the gay liberation movement. Gay and lesbian people were able to begin the process of healing the psychological wounds suffered from the twin rejections by family and society. We talked with each other and tried to get honest. Lives that had been nothing but stolen glances began to bloom. We have made ourselves more whole by this process.

Learning to talk together has not been easy for leather and SM people for exactly the same reasons that it was hard for lesbians and gay men to learn to talk together in the '50s and '60s. You see, kinky people, like gay people, are only supposed to *do it* in secret, in private, in shame, in fear, in self-loathing, and most of all, in silence. And so we did. For a very long time. Until now.

Let's Get Real

"Sacred cows make the best hamburger"

—Overheard

Much to the surprise of many who do not share our particular interests, we Sexual Frontiersmen do think about relationships about as often as, say, our vanilla gay brethren. Some people I know believe that leather men don't enter relationships as often as vanilla gay men. But I certainly have the impression that relationships and how to form them are on our minds a lot, especially in the face of AIDS.

It will be my intention in this space to share with you both my clinical and personal insights into some of the issues and problems that men pursuing the SM lifestyle or SM sexualities encounter as we make our way into the relationships in which we become involved.

Currently, I am a licensed psychotherapist in private practice. Most of my reading, research, writing and public speaking has had SM as its focus. In short, SM has long since become an obsession for me. I consider myself, therefore, blessed. Fate might have chosen any number of boring preoccupations for me, but I was spared!

In my capacity as a therapist, I have spent many hours talking with kinky gay men about a wide variety of issues, including their relationships. Naturally, during the course of so many hours of talk, patterns began to reveal themselves. My hope is that in telling you what I have learned, you will look at your relationships with a fresh perspective, and perhaps come to a way of thinking about them that you may find more workable than before.

"Workable!" What the hell does he mean by that?

41

I mean, does it work for you, or against you? Is it part of the solution, or part of the problem? Does the relationship add to everyone's life, or not? Is the screwing you're getting worth the screwing you're getting?

I had to laugh when Anthony F. DeBlase, then publisher of *Drummer* magazine, suggested I consider writing a column on relationships for his magazine. For years I've had a suppressed desire to bomb their offices! Many of you readers have the experience and sophistication to know that *Drummer* has been primarily a fantasy magazine. But I know from my experience as a therapist that many readers of pornography have tried to pattern their relationships (and sometimes their lives) after the stories they have read, mostly in *Drummer*, occasionally with disastrous results.

This happens most often among younger guys who have just stumbled across the scene and felt a deep resonance within themselves. In the course of trying to respond to these feelings, they soon come across *Drummer* and commonly report that it was like finding the Motherlode. That is, until they went out in search of _____!

Well, needless to say, most of these newcomers have some pretty unreal notions about who they want to marry. And for good reason. The role models in SM fantasy stories, for both Tops and bottoms are more like icons than real people. They don't live real lives. For the most part, they populate worlds where no one works or gets sick or has parents or professional reputations to deal with; where no one has emotional hang-ups, fears, weaknesses, or feelings of being trapped or insecure.

Young people in particular, but also large numbers of the not so young, need role models, of course. Role models somehow tell us how to be what it is we think we want to be. And for those just coming into the scene, the sight of men in leather can be so intimidating that they often just plain don't talk to anyone. Magazines seem instantly more accessible and more controllable. They appear to offer the novice the kind of intimate, insider-type information that he craves in order to give form to those powerful feelings he has banging around in his head and his shorts.

Unfortunately, such a person is not always experienced enough (just in life, let alone the leather scene) to distinguish between probable fantasy and possible reality. These early feelings have a funny way of acting like a template or yardstick against which the validity of later feelings will be measured. I remember so well the experience of seeing my first Tom of Finland drawings, icons of hyper-masculinity, exaggerated to titillate. I have never truly recovered at some level: some part of me compares all men with those internalized images...and with predictably unfortunate results. Stories can work the same way.

In fact, when it comes to role models for SM relationships, the one-handed stories we read often do not even suggest that relationships are possible. With the occasional exception of some stories of wealthy super-masters and their slaves, such as John Preston's infamous "Mister Benson" serial in *Drummer*, one could easily conclude from the available fiction that SM relationships just don't happen. When I came out into the SM/leather scene (the Earth was still cooling) it was a common saying that SM relationships could not and did not last. SM couples who had been together even a few years were spoken of in reverent and respectful terms.

As I began to meet couples who were in the SM scene and was allowed to slowly learn about how their relationships really functioned, I saw that they bore no resemblance to anything that I had ever read about in the underground world of SM publications. It turned out that, for the most part, what makes for good fantasy did not look much like anyone's reality.

The reason, of course, is that one does not live by fantasy alone. As it happens, we do not live by reality alone, either. Typically, the couples that report feeling good about their involvements are those in which the partners together have created a blending of fantasy and reality or, at least, a way to ease the transition back and forth between the two.

By now I have counseled many couples who have struggled mightily in their efforts to achieve this blending of fantasy and reality in their lives. There are no models for how to do it except, perhaps, for those particular couples themselves. Since there are so very many ways to be involved in the SM scene, there is, therefore, no one correct way to do it. But there are some ways that don't seem to work well as far as I can tell.

Couples (triples? quartets too!) in which anyone consistently tries to press the relationship into a fantasy mold that is not shared by the other partner(s) commonly experience troubles, which usually express themselves first somewhere in the sex.

When these people turn up in the therapy room, my usual diagnosis is "Porn-itis." The condition is usually correctable unless there are widely variant values or attitudes about what the relationship should be. Quite often I discover that a partnership was formed and agreed upon before any such joint exploration of ideas and attitudes ever happened. Such exploration usually is not considered hot, you see. So it often doesn't happen until there is a problem.

A relationship has to be written by both Top and bottom as they get to know each other, not lifted out of some hot story. Tops are not mind readers. Some are frighteningly intuitive, but very few are psychic. Bottoms should not expect their minds to be read unless they come complete with an owner's manual. Few do. Many Tops also enjoy projecting the facade that they are mind readers, but they invite trouble when they do.

My point here is simply that no matter how valuable fantasy material is, from whatever source, it offers little of substance to a partnership in need of practical day-to-day operational strategy.

I seem to recall an article somewhere in which Fred Halsted, a Top, pointed out to readers that his bottom/lover of many years (Joey) took care of their auto maintenance, while Fred himself was better at doing the housework (or something like that). I remember being struck by the paradoxical beauty of their arrangement, and I doubt it was copied from any story they had either read or written. The flexibility to be real, and not be bound by stereotyped fiction is a common theme in all the long-term relationships that I have been privileged to become acquainted with.

In fact, there is a lot to say for the slow, cards on the table approach to building a relationship. It allows both Top and bottom to get down to a little reality before dabbling in the fantasy. Thus the blending process can start at the beginning of a relationship, and not be scrambled together when the fantasy founders on the rocks of reality.

And think about this: with our understanding of ritual, leathermen can have a lot more fun with the mating process than perhaps anyone on the planet! For instance, a Top who orchestrates a courtship can enable both himself and his bottom to become familiar with each others' needs, wants and points of view. Honesty is vital. Tops who dangle the promise of sex like a carrot can create sweet tension if they are sincere, but can damage their bottoms and their reputations if they are not.

A Top and bottom who play their cards honestly can steadily gain each others' trust and friendship. And the kind of relationship, and the sex, that can blossom in an open, trusting exchange can be exquisite. Honesty and reality will also protect the interests and feelings of both partners as they move on in or out of the relationship.

Outside, Looking In?

I want to go over some ideas about your relationship with your self. It's important because, after all, you are your only constant companion.

Besides, developing a healthy relationship with all the parts of yourself places you in a better position to have healthy relationships with others. Most of all, I am concerned that many of us have painful relationships with our sexual selves—let me explain.

When SM and leather themes first began to emerge from the mists of my own adolescent horniness, I was scared by them. As I began to discover the world of leathermen, I felt both excited by it and worried about myself. If I were to explore my real desires, I feared that I would somehow be destroyed by them.

I can remember the vague dread that there might be some hidden point past which I could never return to the vanilla world. I would be swept away into some lifestyle that I could not control. It was awful. It was made worse by the fact that I could tell no one about these inclinations or the fears that went with them. I was excited, scared and isolated. The world of SM/leather was like an accident: I couldn't look at it, and I couldn't look away either.

My experience is not unique; I know that there are many people who also feel trapped somewhere between their desire for this sexuality and their fear of it.

By now, I have had the chance both in and out of the therapy room to spend time exploring the issues that surround people's fears about the SM scene. Several general themes have emerged.

First and foremost, it seems that many guys with SM/leather interests are loaded with shame about having them. The shame may come from the belief that it is wrong to enjoy yourself too much, or to be too much different from everyone else. It may also come from the notion that there may be something evil or Satanic about SM/leather sexuality. Some feel that it is shameful to do sexual things with equipment—people is okay, objects are not.

Our recognition that we are *perverts* carries with it the feeling that we have made a shameful mistake in our lives that we must now hide. American society places high value on innocence for some reason. Other societies value experience, ours does not. Therefore, anyone who knows too much about sex is considered sleazy and thus not desirable. So we grow up with the understanding that it is okay to know about suckfuck, but not much more. Other men fear that just thinking about SM/leather sex will mark them somehow, and others will know they are sleazy. The secret will be out.

As males, many of us are following an old straight script that says we are better to settle down with a virgin (or as close as we can get) after we have sown our "wild oats." Some guys go out and get lots of sexual experience, then must downplay it so our potential partner is not scared by our "wild" past.

Some make it okay for themselves to have had their "wild" past by feeling shame about it now. "It's all in the past—I am (like) a virgin again."

Social rules say that straight is better than gay. The rules also say that vanilla is better than kinky. So there is hiding. And a part of us is cut off from ourselves.

When we reject a natural part of ourselves, we damage our self concept, and our confidence in our ability to have happy relationships is undermined. American social pressure to conform is strong. Officially, we are proud of our melting pot image. Our actual behavior as a nation, however, reveals that we do not tolerate diversity. So there is a strong inclination to hide our differentness. In other cases, the individual who is different may wish to have his "uniqueness" removed. So therapists hear, "I am gay, can you make me straight?" Or, "I am kinky, can you make me 'normal'?"

Society, through our parents, uses shame to pressure us into being (or wanting to be) just like everybody else. Most often, the shame that we feel over our differentness is really just an internal reflection of social values that come from outside. In other words, we feel shame because we think we are supposed to feel it. But it does not belong to us. It is what they want us to feel.

The freedom to be different and feel okay about it must be fought for.

Another fear that plagues us as we come out into the SM/leather world is the fear that we are going to be harmed by pursuing these desires. Often we fear physical harm, but many also fear some undefined psychological or spiritual harm. This was my biggest concern when I was 19 and just at the edge of this stuff.

Fortunately, no one lied to me then by trying to tell me that harm—all sorts—was impossible. My intuition had been right about the scene; one could come to some harm in various ways. Stories reached my ears about a very few guys who had been injured, some seriously. Others got lost in the stew of sex and drugs that I knew was swirling around out there. I could tell that it was not all a bed of roses.

Still the magic called me. I began to search out mentors—teachers who could instruct me in navigating a course toward the experiences I wanted without crashing psychologically, physically, emotionally or spiritually. I found them and they taught me, just as they will teach you if you seek them out.

If you try to find your way in the SM/leather scene by yourself, you are doing it the hard way—there is no need. There are now over 200 organizations available to help you and teach you in this country and at least half that number overseas. We now have numerous publications that provide a wealth of information that was not available 20 years ago.

For those of you who feel called to this sexuality, the worst thing you can do is remain isolated in your own fear and shame. The accidents that do happen in the scene usually happen to loners who can't or won't connect to a support system or network of like minded folks for guidance and fellowship. There is now a tribe of Leatherfolk, and it cuts across the lines of gay/straight, male/female, rich/poor, old/young. If you fail to use the tribe's resources for dealing with the shame and fear, you will just hurt and hide longer. Is that really what you want to do with your time?

Let's Not Take The Olde Guard Judges Too Seriously

"If it ain't fun, you ain't doin' it right."

—The Mistress Carolyn

As if SM relationships weren't already complex enough, many of you who are relationship oriented must, at some point, come to terms with the ever present problem of purism. I refer to the need some folks have to make judgments as to whether your relationship is a "true SM relationship" or if you are a "true Master" or a "true masochist" or a "real slave" or "really into the scene."

Sometimes, it seems as if a great conclave had been held somewhere at which time standards for perfection were somehow agreed upon (imagine that!). One would think that a group of people at that gathering were selected as Judges, selected on the basis of some sort of erotico-ideological purity to enforce ideals of SM correctness. Over the years, the letters printed in *Drummer* bear this out. Recently, there was yet another letter from yet another slave acting as Judge regarding the bottom correctness of a person he had never even met.

As a therapist, I see plenty of unpleasant fallout when people in relationships, or wanting them, try to fit themselves into two-dimensional ideals. For example, one purist ideal suggests that a "true slave" obeys his master's every command. None of those Judges out there had to sit with me in the therapy room as I counseled a young man, who, earnestly wanting to prove to a Top that he was slave material, got himself arrested for following an order that was irresponsible.

There is also some notion among the purist Judges that so

51

called "true" Masters and/or Tops never switch or go under, or do otherwise "bottom" things. Certainly some of the Judges frown when Tops tell their bottoms to pinch tits or slap ass. And the Judges go positively crazy when Tops switch their keys to enter a relationship as a bottom.

Likewise, bottoms who come out as Tops are often not taken seriously by other bottoms until a decent (?) interval of time has passed; he is Judged to be unpredictable or not authentic or some such. There are even Judges who have put Tops down for kissing bottoms.

It is at once amusing, ironic and depressing to recognize that some in the SM/leather scene employ the same oppressive you-are-not-OK tactics to standardize SM behaviors that non-SM people use to "normalize" us. One would think that we get enough of that judgmentalism from outside the SM community; surely we don't have to do that to each other.

The last time I checked, I noticed that there was no single right way to do anything. There seem to be lots of ways to be a real slave, or Master, or rock star, or stock broker or anything else. Relationships are no different. The definitive rule book has not and cannot be written. The range of human variability is too wide. SM and SM relationships will not be boxed in by the Judges no matter how much they may pontificate.

Only you are qualified to assess the correctness of a relationship that you are in. After all, only you could possibly possess the information about how the relationship feels. There are lots of people out there both gay and straight who have so called "correct" relationships, and who also just happen to be miserable as hell. The better litmus test is whether or not the relationship works for you, and not whether it conforms to someone else's ideal.

Let me illustrate. I have seen two Masters each having dinner with their slaves at two separate tables in the same restaurant. Naturally, the waiters at each table placed menus before both Master and slave. At one table, the slave picked up his menu and gave it, unopened, to his Master. The Master ordered dinner for both and later, paid the check. At the other table, the Master picked up his menu, unopened, and handed it to his slave. The slave ordered dinner for both, and later, it was he who paid the check. We see at once that each Master and slave have worked out this situation very differently. Though the form of each relationship appears opposite, apparently, both are correct for the people involved.

In SM relationships, as in life, things are not always what they seem. This fact is what makes Judging relationships both difficult and silly. I know Tops who order their bottoms to wear white sneakers into leather bars as a humiliation—does that mean the bottoms aren't "really into the scene?" I also know of very sadistic Tops who are not into leather at all, who will go into bars in casual wear with their leathered out bottoms and proceed to work their submissives over in public. According to the old guard stereotypes, it looks like the preppie ought to be the bottom, or even vanilla, but then, in this instance, it turns out otherwise. It is still true what they say about books and their covers.

If for some reason, it works for a bottom to dress on the left, then who is to challenge? Perhaps he wants to fend off novice Tops that night, or needs to switch for the first time in a while. If Tops want rings in their whatevers, then that must be their prerogative. Who says that it's the Top in relationships who has the best judgment in all matters? We all know that in some things bottoms may have some superior ability that wise Tops will not want to waste just to prove who is boss.

Your relationships in kinky life must be free to take whatever form is needed to meet your needs and the needs of your partner(s). That form must also be free to evolve as you grow and change. You who are willing and able to be that free and flexible deserve praise for your honesty, love, commitment, and imagination. The Judges who shake their fingers at those who may shape their relationships to the beat of a different drummer are simply revealing the choices they make for themselves. Variation can add richness to the scene, and we will do better to encourage experimentation and diversity than to scold those who leave the stereotypes behind in their own

53

search for happiness and satisfaction in the world of SM relationships.

Blindman's Bluff Hurts Too Much

Previously, I suggested that one-handed reading isn't very helpful to those of you who want some clues about how to put together some sort of SM relationship for yourselves. Now, I am here to tell you that there is a bountiful storehouse chock full of clues just waiting to help you. It's in a place where you may not have thought to look—inside yourself.

Therapists would have to do a lot less work repairing partnerships that have gone out of kilter, if people would do their "homework" before they get involved. This is especially true in SM relationships, because, I believe, they are more complex dynamically that non-SM relationships. In short, I am suggesting that relationships will often run more smoothly if they have been prepared for.

A helpful first step is to get honest about what you really want, from both the kinky and non-kinky aspects of your involvements. In addition to all the other considerations that go with non-SM relationships (Is he/she attractive? Do they need to be? etc.), there are the SM issues. Ask yourself some questions:

To what degree do you need to shape your life around the exploration of your sexuality? Some will want lover-type relationships with varying degrees of SM stuff whenever both are horny. These are relationships with SM in them.

Others will prefer to live lives with SM as the relationship. Consider life in a cage, if you will? Or what about being a full-time Master or Mistress with various sorts of slaves at your beck and call? Such full-time involvements are indeed possible, but developing them in the real world can be a slow and difficult process.

At the other end of the spectrum from the full-time Dominants/submissives are those who want SM relationships only in fantasy, and have no thought of actualizing their desires. The point is that there are lots of ways to weave SM into your relationships, but the shape of the relationships must emerge from honest self-examination.

The subject of love in an SM relationship is too complex to be handled reasonably here. For now, consider at least whether or not you need to love, or be loved by, your SM counterpart in order to have a satisfying relationship. Some people don't want a kinky lover and prefer to get their SM needs met outside their primary or romantic involvements. The opposite works for others. Their SM relationship is primary, and there are lovers or affairs of the heart "outside," to speak.

What do you need? John's offering of his submission and suffering to a Top is an "I love you" message in and of itself. He will not suffer at the hand of any man for whom he cannot feel love. Richard, a sadist, can't hurt anyone he does love. His equally sadistic friend, Tom, believes that he wastes himself when he hurts those for whom he feels nothing romantic. Clearly, there are many angles to this issue, and lots of opportunities for a mismatch if one is not scrupulously honest first with oneself.

There is in all of this a presumption of experience—not even necessarily a lot, but some is essential. It's hard to know how you really feel about Paris until you go there yourself. You can form a provisional opinion based on what you read, see in films and photos, or hear in the stories of friends who've been there. SM relationships as they really operate are almost never filmed, photographed or written about. Increasingly, however, people are starting to talk about them some, and this can help supplement your own experience in deciding what sort of configuration might be right for you next.

It is equally useful to think about the distinctions between words like slave, masochist, and submissive; or Master, Mistress, sadist, and dominant as they may apply to yourself. I don't mean to suggest that these words are pigeonholes into which you should place yourself. Rather, they are words that describe evolving and dynamic processes that can give shape to your thinking about your sexuality and where you might want to go with it.

A person's tastes often evolve during his erotic lifetime. What may have been true for him two years ago may have changed by now. Research has suggested that when it comes to exotic sexualities, most people "go both ways." That is to say they switch or think about switching polarities from time to time between their dominant and submissive selves. I'll refer to these people as "switches."

For functional switches, i.e. those who move back and forth between Top and bottom comfortably on their own timetables, the act of switching can be caused by several things. Some switch because they like to. Others do so because they want access to partners irrespective of the other person's preference. Others switch as an act of love to satisfy a lover's need. Whatever the reason, check yourself out. Do you switch? Why? With the same partner? In the same scene? Will you want a relationship with another switch? Will you only switch outside a relationship? Take notes on yourself. Successful relationships result from hard work. Doing some work with yourself will help with the relationship you're in, or prepare you for the one you want.

What about your real feelings concerning SM and drugs and alcohol? How do they affect your ability to play both safely and wisely? Will you rule out relationship candidates if their thinking about drugs is much different from your own?

Is public or semi-public playing something you like a lot or not at all? Do you socialize in the SM world? Do you need your partner to do so as well? Where do you stand with regard to marks on the body, both temporary and permanent? The range of possibilities is wide here, from rope and whip marks, shaving, body-painting and even sunburn on the temporary side, to tattoos, piercings, scarification and branding on the permanent. Are these marks trophies or blemishes in your eyes?

What about being involved with more than one person at a time, either in a scene or perhaps as a member of a family of three or four? Do you want to have a stable of slaves or a harem of submissives? Do you dream of being owned by a group of Masters or used by a group of Mistresses? Do you want to make these fantasies into day-to-day realities, or are you content to pull them out in horny moments?

Recently, I have become aware of no fewer than seven SM relationships involving three or more persons. None were similar to any other in either structure or function. Although such possibilities abound, any relationship necessarily begins with individuals. The more information you have about yourself, the better equipped you are to have a relationship with yourself first and then others. Getting to know your sexuality is tough enough when it's not an unusual one. It's harder when it's exotic, and there's no support from any majority or minority social institutions to assist you in your self-examination.

But look inward we must. The blindman's bluff approach to relationships just doesn't work very well. In that game, you make your choice of partners with a blindfold on, i.e. you don't look at him to see who he is, and you don't look at yourself to see who you are. Who can be surprised at the results?

Men Who Like To Switch: Treasures And Tribulations

Friends and clients alike have often commented to me about the difficulty of finding a good "fit" with another person. Even when they connect with someone special and work out the other relationship issues, finding the SM fit is often elusive.

Those men who like to switch back and forth between Top and bottom make this complaint more often than the men who express their sexuality in only one style. In the old days, switches were sort of second class citizens in the SM world—they were often seen as indecisive. The more accurate view is that they have the freedom to express all sides of their personalities in a sexual way. In a sense, the switch may have several sexual "personalities" to "choose from" when he gets horny.

I have found that one useful way of thinking about the range of "SM personalities" is to think in terms of relevant themes that characterize particular sexual styles. So far, three major themes have come to my attention. They are: dominant and submissive, sadistic and masochistic, and aggressive and passive. Expressed graphically they look like this:

```
Dominance ——I   vanilla  I—— Submission
  Sadistic ——I    zone    I—— Masochistic
Aggressive ————O———— Passive
```

So, for example, I have a friend who is an aggressive submissive, but not at all masochistic. I know others who I would usually describe as submissive sadists who are passive (suggestible in this case). A friend in New York (and another in Los Angeles, come to think of it) is an aggressive, dominant masochist. Another is a dominant sadist, but neither aggressive

59

nor passive. Adversarial SM is the stuff that happens between aggressive sadists and aggressive masochists who are both dominant.

The stereotyped Top is all those things on the left, while the stereotyped bottom is all those things on the right. Most folks are various configurations of these themes, and, importantly, they usually change from day to day or even moment to moment. This changing is very healthy from a psychological point of view, because it allows for flexible responses to changing situations.

For example, one day I might start to *feel* aggressive, sadistic and dominant as hell. I might function in this Top way for quite a while before I start feeling some change—perhaps I might still feel sadistic later, but more passive. Still later, I might feel the need to submit to a Top myself.

The tough part for relationships comes when the Switch feels that he must find the one person who is the perfect counterpart for all of his sexual personalities. For some, the problem may be like trying to find the restaurant that has all your favorite dishes on the menu, each prepared by world class chefs.

So I hear remarks in my office like, "Everything is perfect with us except that he does not want to top me," or "Sometimes, I don't want to play with the masochist I have, but I do want to play with the slave I don't have." "I am crazy for uniforms, and he hates them." "He won't play outdoors no matter what."

Here are some issues to consider about relationships for those who switch. Just how much overlap in sexualities do you require in a partner? Remember that few of us come to relationships with full sexual development—we learn from our partners about new things. Assessing someone's capacity to grow sexually is not easy; it takes time and patience. Are you a good teacher? Is it easy for you to learn about new sexual things?

If you discover that there are some sexual things that you don't have in common, how will you feel about going outside

60

the relationship to get those needs met? And what if he wants to go outside for the same reason? Studies of gay male relationships show that usually by the end of the fifth year, the men have made some provisions for outside erotic experiences. Researchers have discovered that most gay men do not define fidelity in terms of sexual exclusivity as heterosexuals more commonly do. It is almost as though gay men understand the futility of trying to own another person's sexual attention.

When provisions for outside sexual experiences are made, they must be carefully negotiated with agreed upon rules. Here are some of the types of rules that I have heard about: I never/always want to hear about it; Never in our house (bed); I never/always want to meet him; I always/never want to hear intimate details of the scene; Only when I am (or you are) out of town; I don't want you to do (such and such) with anyone but me; I don't want you to play with them more than once (twice?); I would prefer that you find a regular person to play with. These and other rules may exist singly or with each other.

In general, it is unwise to kiss off something that you like just because your partner isn't into it. (I am not talking about unsafe sexual practices. Those should already have been kissed off!) Doing so causes resentment to build, and sooner or later, you will want your pound of flesh to make up for your *sacrifice*. Look for a way to get your needs met within the relationship first if possible, and outside if not. Talk until it's all talked out. Involve your partner in your thoughts and feelings as you reach your decisions. Until a solution is agreed upon, *both* (all) partners will still have a problem. Unresolved issues in relationships become buried land mines that we can trip on later.

The other important trouble spot has to do with timing. Usually to play, the polarities have to be complementary. For example, when two switches are in a relationship, if they are both feeling Toppy, at the same time, that can be a problem. Same problem exists when each wants to submit to the other.

In working with couples who have this issue, I have found that one useful solution is to encourage the one who gets horny first to send the appropriate cues to the other partner in a effort to influence which buttons get pushed.

Let's say that I'm a switch and want my partner to top me tonight. I might start behaving like the sort of bottom I know he likes. I could sit at his feet after dinner and maybe clean his boots to see if I could turn his Top stuff on. If I wanted to top him, I might serve him dinner on the floor, or tell him what I wanted him to wear or whatever I thought might turn his bottom side on. If these strategies don't work, we could consider striking a deal for the evening. Couples do this, and some know how to make it work.

Some guys choose to get both their Top and bottom needs met in the SM scene by switching back and forth. In some ways, this is an advantage, a bit like having several Tops and several bottoms all rolled into one partner. There are also special challenges, and switches do better when they develop keen sensitivity to the shifts in their own feelings, and act accordingly.

Each of the changes we are talking about can be like a change in sexual and emotional weather. Some men can change their own weather at will. I know bottoms who can switch their own Top stuff on instantly if the right bottom walks into the room. A friend once said, "Show me the man, and I'll tell you what's possible."

Lives have a way of balancing themselves out, and (my opinion now) we probably use SM as a tool with which to achieve those balances on a day-in/day-out basis. My guess is that we all have both dominant and submissive sides. Any Top who has had to knuckle under to a powerful boss knows what I mean. Any slave who has been told to make dinner with no questions also has to learn about his dominant side in order to take charge of the kitchen and make the decisions on his own that will produce a meal. I'll wager that when aggressive drivers see a cop, they get passive real fast. It is all situational.

Few people today will argue with the notion that sexual expression is recreational—that is, re-creation. My view is that the thing we re-create in our lives when we play is balance. I don't think it matters what kind of play we are talking about either—golf or whips.

Three Or More?

Things seem to come in cycles for some reason, and recently, I have received several requests to comment on the special circumstances that tend to come up when so called "group" or multiple relationships are attempted in the context of dominance and submission or SM relationships. I know that group relationships are a subject of interest for many of us partly because fictional stories about them turn up so often, and partly because many of my clients report that erotic fantasies about group relationships have a steady attraction for them. This fascination seems to be interesting to Tops about as often as it is to bottoms, although there is no research to support this observation. So, who can be surprised that some of us sometimes try to make such fantasies real?

Fantasies about group relationships usually come in one (or more) of these configurations: one slave in service to two or more Masters/Mistresses; one Master/Mistress with a stable of submissives; two or more Top/bottom couples who co-habit and play together; and/or a pool of Dominants who ride herd over a dungeon of bottoms. Many writers of SM fiction have titillated us at one time or another with stories based on these models.

Since general society sanctions the standard marital pair, most of our experience with relationships comes from our participation in what is known as the pair bond—we become lovers with one other person. Consequently, most of the group relationships with which I am familiar both in and out of the therapy room began when a Top/bottom couple who identified themselves as "lovers" decided to involve themselves with either another individual or another set of kinky lovers with whom there was a mutual attraction.

Among the relationships of these types I know of, almost without exception, trouble started just about immediately. And it always seems to start in the same way: somebody gets hurt feelings. Either one of the pre-existing lovers starts hurting, or the newcomer does. In either case, typically the hurting one reports his feelings to the other member of the triad with whom he feels the most emotional closeness. This message is then transmitted to the third member by the second.

The hurt feelings usually come up around one or more of the following issues: division of labor; division of time; different income or debt; differences in sexual frequency or activity; differences in schedule; competition for time, intimacy, sex, authority, or affection. In other words, it's all the usual stuff that troubles diads (pronounced, die-adds, meaning standard couples). Making the extra effort to acquire the skills necessary to work these problems out is a huge challenge, and this is the usual reason given for the assertion that multiple relationships are inherently unstable. People are just not up to the challenges offered by these relationships. Most of us somehow sense that we are not up to it, so we don't even try in the first place.

Even when the members of the new multiple relationship are able to work these problems out to everyone's mutual satisfaction, these same issues are likely to come up all over again if a decision is made to add one or more guys to the multiple partnership at some later date. The individuals in most triads are often so exhausted by the effort to stabilize the trio that they become very reluctant to attempt any enlargement of the relationship afterwards. In some cases, the exhaustion leads to the breakup of the triad and either a return to the original diad, a total breakup, or the formation of a new diad. Whatever the end result, emotional wounds are usually suffered by all parties. Such wounds are not easily forgotten.

Having said all that, I must also point out that I know of seven such multiple relationships currently underway that seem to be working well. Three of them are triads, and one of them has seven members (it includes one woman, I might add). As luck would have it, I have been allowed to learn some things about how they happened, some problems that have been overcome, and how. All but one of these began with an original pair and then grew.

What follows are some suggestions which I hope can be helpful for those contemplating such an attempt.

First of all, at the point when both lovers confide to each other that they each have an interest in adding one or more to their original relationship, it seems to be very important that they first talk honestly with each other about *exactly* what sort of configuration each has been thinking about. If it is discovered that their views of a possible triad are similar with respect to roles, living arrangements, sleeping and sexual arrangements, and the other issues mentioned earlier, then their discussions might safely proceed. If they are different in important aspects, they would be well advised to keep their interest at the fantasy level for the duration of their relationship, or until their attitudes change.

If there is general agreement on the important aspects and they decide to proceed, then the couple would be wise to (separately) list what sort of person each thinks might be a workable addition. This list should be written down and include things like the physical, emotional, intellectual, spiritual, erotic, and character attributes of the possible candidate; his life circumstances; goals and aspirations; safer sex guidelines; along with comments about undesirable traits or features of the candidate. Such lists should then be shared with one's partner to determine compatibility. All this is better done before any effort is made to search for a candidate—otherwise, how would they know what sort of person to look for?

Likewise, if a single guy is interested in a multiple relationship, he too would be well advised to spend some time developing such a list while taking great care to be rigorously honest with himself about what he thinks might work best for himself. The message is: its very hard to find something if you don't know what you're looking for.

It is a good idea to develop such a list over time, say, a

month or two, so you can try on the ideas contained in the list in your head. Something that seems like a good idea at first might not after you've thought about it a while. Don't be afraid to change the list as your thinking changes, but stay honest with yourself!

Once you've settled on a package of ideas that you think you can live with, you have essentially two choices: either you can hope to run into the situation you seek with another person or persons, or you can advertise. Yes, advertise. It's the fastest way I know of to communicate with the largest number of people, and it works out more often than not if you handle your responses carefully and honestly and craft a good ad in the first place. The experience of myself and others recommends that you not be willing to compromise on the more important features found on your list.

If fortune smiles on you and you connect with serious and compatible candidates, do your level best when you meet to speak honestly and openly with each other about what everyone needs and what everyone can offer right from the beginning. Failure to do this will only *delay* the onset of problem solving efforts later.

If it turns out that all the lights are green, I suggest that a temporary arrangement be made, say maybe a month or six weeks with an agreement to talk at least weekly about how things are going. What seems to be working out well and what is not will have to be discussed frankly. Such conversations could include reporting any emotional surprises that anyone notices coming up with respect to himself or the others. Perhaps the most important emotional information to share has to do with any fear or anger that pops up.

Whenever possible during such conversations, it is helpful to ask for specific behavior changes from whoever is frightening or annoying. Even if one is not sure what he wants to see change, it can be helpful to offer a guess.

Unless a specific structure with rules for communication is created, it is generally dangerous when one person begins carrying emotional messages *for* someone else to a third person.

Things tend to go more smoothly when messages about feelings are announced to all members of a group relationship at the same time. The group relationship with seven people that I mentioned earlier has a standing rule that hassles are communicated in front of all other members at the same time. This rule keeps everybody up to speed on the state of all the one-on-one relationships at the same time, so that everybody knows how everybody feels about everybody else with the minimum time delay. In a sense, this works out to be a kind of group therapy with one of the uninvolved dominants acting as group facilitator or referee.

Jealousy is a common complaint that all such relationships must come to terms with. It is useful to bear in mind the fact that no person loves in the same way twice nor can they be expected to do so. Furthermore, nowhere is it written that all members of such a relationship must necessarily be in love with each other in order for the relationship to work out well.

At their most basic level, relationships happen between two people or entities at a time. This means that when three become involved, there are really a total of six different relationships: the three between each of the three pairs, and three more between any individual and each of the other pairs. Not included in this list is the relationship one has with one's self.

For triads to survive, all of these relationships must be in relatively good repair at least most of the time. As you might guess, this can be a complicated process to manage, and will require great commitment and effort on everyone's part. But it can be done if everyone has the ability to tell the truth to one's self and others, to listen carefully, and to say what they mean and mean what they say.

Group relationships are not for everyone. In practice, they can offer special rewards and create special problems. They take extra time and lots of energy. Although there is much more to say about all this, the above should give anyone thinking about such relationships more than enough to chew on. I hope that, in time, we will all hear more from those for whom such relationships work, and also from those who have had difficulty.

Only in this way will we be able to profit from the experiences of others who choose this option for themselves.

Master/Slave Relationships: An Overview

"He serves best who serves the servant."

—Thom Magister

In this and the next essay, I want to focus on relationships with prevailing dominant/submissive features, specifically, Master/slave relationships. Obviously, most (if not all) of what I say will be equally applicable to Mistress/slave relationships. You are encouraged to read into my male-male language your own gender combination. Regardless of genders, the subject is the relationship between a confirmed Dominant and a willing submissive. These Master/Mistress-slave relationships are usually seen by their practitioners as the ultimate expression of the dominant/submissive experience.

Put in simple terms, these relationships occur between the identified Master who has a defined authority and specified responsibilities in the relationship, and the identified slave(s) who submit(s) to the will of the Master.

The variation here is wide. When and where? This configuration may only happen at certain times of the day, or on certain days of the week, or in certain rooms, or when certain clothes are worn, or perhaps only in the presence of certain people etc.

Is there more than one way to do it? You bet! Just to give you a feeling for the range of possibilities, I have seen a Master with several slaves. Some slaves have more than one Master. Some slaves have slaves, and some Masters are themselves slaves to yet other Masters. Another slave I know has a lover (mostly vanilla) and a Master as well—each knows and likes the other. And yes, I know of Master/slave involvements that

71

have been ongoing now for many years. The partners have learned to manage the intensity and keep things hot for themselves, mostly through the development of a remarkable degree of honesty.

Written contracts sometimes add an interesting wrinkle—I have seen several. Again, variation is wide. Some Masters have authority in the slave's work place (if the slave works). Some slaves have autonomy when dealing with their family; some not. Finances are not always subject to the Master's will, whereas some Masters require their slave to handle *all* finances. Some Masters outline various levels of submission, with deepest submission, usually very short term, such that the slave does nothing but breathe without instructions.

I have spoken with many guys who have found ecstasy in the Master/slave scene. Most reported to me that they had to explore several different such situations first before they could learn enough about themselves to know what would work for their own particular personalities.

If this is something you have only dreamed about your whole life, look inside yourself to learn what has kept you from trying it out. It is not too much trouble to find your counterpart especially for short term "try it on for size" scenes.

Hot times are to be had over the phone or through the mails. My own first experience came from a stranger whispering softly in my ear one night at some bar in Denver. We talked maybe for 20 minutes, then he left alone. I like to think that it changed us both.

It is unfair to yourself to assume that the relationship in your mind cannot be achieved, at least in part. Remember that not so many years ago, it was impossible for a closeted gay man to even imagine an ongoing relationship with another man.

Likewise, if this is your scene and you find yourself bouncing from one Master/slave situation to another in frustration, perhaps now might be a good time to check out your motivations for wanting this sort of thing in the first place. If you only end up with bad apples, then maybe you need to refine your pickin' skills. It helps to distinguish between what you can tolerate and what you can dream about.

In designing these relationships, one watchword comes from the Mistress Carolyn. Her advice: "If it ain't fun, you ain't doin' it right." I take her to mean that the rituals, rules, responsibilities, and restrictions that are incorporated into the relationship must be a turn on for everyone, or else, they won't survive for long.

One thing that I have noticed about these relationships is the great extent to which they have been negotiated. Unless these relationships are a perfect sexual and emotional fit from the beginning (and when does that happen?), they will have to be carefully negotiated. In each such relationship that I have happened to learn about, tremendous effort had been made to carefully outline the extent of the Master's authority and responsibility and the extent of the slave's submission.

The durability of these relationships is often determined by the success of the negotiations, and the ability of the partners to remain interesting to each other. Very often, the "divorce clock" starts ticking when one or both start to get bored for long stretches.

In some Master/slave relationships, a man's entry into the position of "slave" represents an "I love you, I trust you" message. Here, a Master's acceptance of a slave represents the complementary "I love you, I trust you" message. It will almost certainly take each of them some time to define for themselves just what "I love you, I trust you" actually means. Right at first, they probably won't know themselves.

It is these definitions of love and trust that will determine how the relationship functions, and how long it will last. It is quite normal for these definitions to change with time.

For example, "I love you, I trust you" for the first week of the relationship may mean, "I love the way you lick my boots, and I trust you not to scuff them up." By the end of the first month, it may have changed to include "I love how I feel when we are together, and I trust you not to lie to me about important things."

By the end of the first year, the definition may include, "I love you because you reveal me to myself, and I trust you with my heart." After more time (?), "I love you 'cause you know me, I trust you with my Self." Whatever. Nigel Kent once said, "If you beat the shit out of a man, he will learn all about you." Certainly, the same is true whether you are the owned or the owner—he will eventually find out who you really are.

My clinical work has taught me that there are also Master/slave relationships in which love is not necessarily part of the equation. In these, the dynamic can be one in which the slave says, consciously or not, "I will take certain risks (usually including obedience) because I enjoy doing so," while the Master says "I will accept the risks of responsibility and your obedience until I loose interest in doing so."

Any of numerous sorts of Master/slave relationships can also include any variety of physical SM practices. Of course, these are optional depending on the tastes of the men involved. At various points in the relationship, the partners may agree to "switch off" the Master/slave process, and leave the physical SM switches on, or vice versa. Usually, either partner can switch something off, but it takes both to turn the switches on again.

For example, a partnership used to having a playroom may switch off the physical SM parts when the room is "out of commission" for some reason or other (Mother's visit?). There are men who refuse to play except in a playroom and won't until their's is set up in a just purchased house, for example. Yet, they can remain Master and slave in the meantime.

Or, perhaps a slave has just broken a leg and feels humiliated by the "uselessness" of his condition. Masters in these situations have been known to "switch off" the Master/slave process, and content themselves with exploring the bondage possibilities presented by the cast. Other Masters in the same situation might do just the opposite. Perhaps they are amused by the sight of a man serving dinner on crutches, who knows? So-o-o-o-o many ways to do this scene...

These relationships can be very rewarding or they can be hell. Mixtures of both are not unknown. My observation has been that the hellish variety is more likely when the men are not honest with themselves first, and with their partner second. Secretly held feelings usually find their expression somewhere in the relationship, and will have to be dealt with sooner or later. In the next essay, I want to go somewhat deeper into the issues that come up for guys into the Master/slave scene in the hope that I can save people some time and unwanted pain.

Master/Slave Relationships: Warnings

"Hail, fellow, well met,
All dirty and wet:
Find out, if you can,
Who's master, who's man."

—Swift, *My Lady's Lamentation*

In the previous essay, I made some more or less introductory remarks about the Master/slave scene, and now I want to try to expand that discussion in the hope of helping folks avoid the quicksand pits that can plague these relationships.

Kinky people are just like other people in that everyone tries to avoid unwanted pain. Relationships that don't work cause pain (not the desirable kind, either), and are, therefore, to be avoided when possible. What follows are some ideas about things I have learned both in and out of the therapy room that might make these relationships more satisfying for you.

First of all, I want to point out that people often tend to bring whatever mess they may have made in their lives to the relationship in hopes that the relationship or the partner will fix whatever is wrong. This is generally a recipe for disaster, because almost nobody is honest about this agenda in the first place—the "he will fix it" agenda is kept secret.

It is kept a secret because somewhere down deep, we know that it's weird to start relationships with the expectation that all we need is the right lover to make things feel good in our lives. It is a romantic idea that is often supported in movies and books and fairy tales. So we don't tell him that he is our (secret) dream man because we know that he would laugh at us, and tell us to get lost if he found out.

The other reason it is kept secret is that we sense the danger of revealing just how much we are depending on him, counting on him to make things better in our lives. We are usually willing for him to find this out gradually as he gets committed to the relationship, but not too much truth at first, Please! Conventional mythology has it that all this is a bottom strategy, but, believe me, Tops do it too, but are even less honest about it.

In either case, slaves and Masters both tend to have fewer troubles in relationships when they have each prepared for the experience first by doing any needed housecleaning in their own lives. If you are planning to sell your car, you know that you will do better if you clean it up first, and do at least the minor repairs—same with your life when you are looking for a relationship. Do what you can to maximize your assets and minimize your personal liabilities before you go a-courtin'.

A common Master complaint is that slaves handle their own money poorly, and may arrive in the relationship with credit card problems or other credit entanglements. It can be useful for Masters to discover how a bottom had planned to deal with the situation before he became a slave. In treatment it often comes out that slave's fantasy was that, someday, a Master would appear riding a big black Harley and make all those nasty debts go away.

A new slave I know had the shock of getting a call from his new Master who had been arrested and was in jail. It seems that there had been a slew of unpaid traffic tickets which the Top had refused to deal with since he thought them all unjust. The slave knew nothing of this, but began to wonder just how much responsibility he could expect from his new Master. They entered treatment together...where all hidden stuff began to emerge.

You will feel much better about yourself going into a relationship if you accept responsibility for how your life is, and take steps to clear the mess out first. There are fewer land mines to stumble on that way.

If you are already in a relationship, do what you can to remain or become an interesting person to be with. Take your own interests seriously, and develop them. Relationships are less likely to get stale when both partners are constantly turning on to themselves and growing. Then, there is always something new to bring into the relationship, and to share with your partner. Every time he sees you are into something interesting, he will be reminded how smart he is to have chosen you to share this time in life with.

One Master I know required his slave to get conversant with impressionist art, because a trip through the great museums of Europe had been planned. The slave became well versed on most of the art they were to see, and a new interest was born for both of them.

Masters and slaves are more interesting to each other when they have time to enjoy their relationship. Those guys who dream of having (or being) slaves, but travel 9 days a week or work 10 hours a day and then do volunteer work before going to some rehearsal, aren't yet taking their dreams seriously enough to make space in their lives for this or any other kind of relationship for that matter.

Masters, once you do make time in your life for a slave, think about it a whole lot before you go shopping, because slaves come in all different kinds of slavery. Few slaves are able or willing to change styles very much. After all, everyone's cock pretty much has a mind of it's own. You can reshape the sexuality of slaves, but it is damn hard work, it takes patience, and it may not work anyway.

It is much better to shop for a Buick if that is what you want rather than get a tractor and then try to rebuild it. This means that it will save much time and anguish if you are willing to interview prospective partners to see if his version of being a slave matches up with your own.

Getting a new boat without thinking first how it might fit into your life is stupid and expensive—the same is true of slaves. A horizontal Master may change his mind about wanting a slave when he cums and gets up out of bed, and then looks at his life while standing up.

One problem that comes up often is that some slaves looking to connect to a Master like to pretend that they, themselves, have few needs or wants beyond that of serving their Master. That might be true for an evening, or a weekend, or even an occasional week. But, since slaves come out of a non-slave society, they also have non-slave needs that run deep, like music, education, travel, and other things they have gotten used to throughout their lives. They often need some social contact, and (heaven forbid) they will need some freedom now and then too. Never mind what kind—they will let you know soon enough—besides, it varies from slave to slave. Try to find out first.

Any candidate slave who asserts that he has no needs of his own should be asked the same questions *after* he has cum. Unfortunately, many slaves kid themselves into believing that they have no other needs than to serve. Masters, proceed with caution!

Slaves' rigid adherence to the idea that they wish only to serve can produce questions like, "Just which three eggs did you want me to scramble, Sir?" or "Just how did you want me to clean the toilet (feed the dog, wash the car, drive to the grocery store, pay the bills, design the new addition, organize our trip to Italy)?". A slave can make being a Master hell when he wants to.

Now, there are some Masters who appreciate this degree of consultation, but work in the therapy room has revealed that they are few and far between. Most aspiring slaves will usually have to realize that Master only wants submission when it pleases Master, and that, at other times, slaves are expected to be on auto pilot.

Masters do not help the situation when they are unclear about just which decisions are and are not to be brought to Him for consultation. Masters who change their minds frequently about these things don't make slavery a joy either.

Just as in Rome, sometimes the most valued slaves tend to be the ones that can take over responsibilities from their

Masters. Many modern Masters, like ancient ones, like their leisure, and appreciate not having to go to the dry cleaners to pick up suits or write out the checks at the end of the month.

Those more rare Masters who want more complete responsibility are usually delighted to find that the bottom has made a mess of his life, because Master can then mount his White (black?) Charger and save the day for the helpless bottom, make him a slave, and live happily ever after.

Those who desire slavery with no decisions (a common fantasy) are really asking that a Master become like a parent to a very young child, say about 3 or 4 years old. I have nothing against infantilism, but "slaves" will do better if they make this particular fantasy known up front. Otherwise, the slave will get resentful the first time Master requires slave to act independently.

Some Masters love this degree of responsibility for each and every move a slave makes, but these are the more rare kind. If your version of how to be a slave includes no decision making, you will have to search for a Master very carefully so as not to mislead candidate Masters.

These scenarios often work great for a while—usually until Master gets bored or gets ill or is seriously injured or somehow dies. Any of these events will generate a crisis because the dependent slave suddenly realizes that his Master is only a man, and that all men must sometimes be dependent on others. This sort of (dependent) slave can fall completely apart in times of crisis.

Highly dependent slaves report feeling very threatened when there is a possibility that they may have to suddenly become responsible again—especially if they must become responsible in some way *for* their Master. The reversal in roles can spook them into running away, and has.

Masters into this scene with highly dependent slaves will need to understand that they must make provisions for the slave in case of incapacity or death. They must also make *outside* provisions for themselves in the event that the slave cannot tolerate the transition back to responsibility. This might mean establishing a network of friends who can take up the slack in times of illness or other disability.

Highly dependent slaves are usually higher maintenance than independent slaves. Masters must therefore get honest with themselves *before* they make their selection.

It is as irresponsible to put a guy on a highly dependent slave trip out on the street as it is to buy a very young puppy one day and then put it out on the street after you decide you don't like changing the training papers any more. Therapists and friends will have to help the rejected slave pick up the pieces of his life again, and it will be a long time before he trusts a Top again.

Bottoms who desire a position as a slave need to realize that Masters too, come in all sizes and shapes both inside and out. Some Masters are dominant during sexual play, but not at other times. Others are dominant at other times, but not during sexual play. Some Masters will assert their privilege to play with other slaves while expecting exclusivity from their number one slave. Some will want to add other slaves.

Slaves also need to understand that not all Masters are into the physical SM scene, and that the sex may be conventional. In the Master/slave scene, most of the stimulation and excitement usually comes from the control part of the relationship. (In physical SM, most of the excitement usually comes through the physical stimulations first, and the dominance and visuals second.)

All this means that Masters need to interview slaves, and that (yes, that's right) slaves need to interview Masters. Many Masters get stuffy and outraged at the suggestion that they should submit themselves to being interviewed by a "lowly" slave.

Their upsetness usually lasts about as long as it takes for them to count the number of slaves they have gone through, or the number of weeks they have spent licking their wounds after a relationship crashed and burned. (Yes, Masters get wounded too.)

Slaves, too, have a hard time facing their responsibility to get enough information from prospective Masters to know whether to pursue the man or cut loose.

This brings us to an interesting paradox (the world of SM is filled with 'em). The dominant Master will need to carefully set his dominance aside to allow the candidate slave to gather the information he will need to decide to surrender to this particular Master. Likewise, the submissive slave will have to set his own submission aside and take a somewhat more dominant and responsible position in order to gather the information needed to determine if a "fit" might be possible.

I don't mean for this process to sound so formal—it isn't. This stuff happens during the relaxed moments of the courtship—over breakfast, while driving to a film, maybe over coffee. But unless the men make time to see if their ideas about Master/slave issues mesh, they are leaving it all up to chance. That is unwise.

When Partners Play Together

*"Remember, if you don't give it to him,
he will find it somewhere else."*

—Mr. Kane

One of the more common complaints that I hear from SM partners who have relationship troubles is that they often have a hard time getting down to a scene. Actually, when you think about it, it is not surprising that a relationship with troubles would include problems in the playroom. Quite frequently, troubles in the relationship will express themselves in the sexuality of the partnership. Likewise, when the relationship issues get resolved, bingo, the sexual stuff will often clear up almost as if by magic.

My inquiries about these difficulties usually reveal that the problems began when the courtship phase of the relationship ended, and the commitment phase began. This may happen because scenes start to count for more in the context of a relationship than when they are just "romps in the playroom" with a hot stranger.

A scene between two people in a healthy relationship functions as a bonding agent. It's one of the glues that helps hold things together. When partners play together, the scene becomes a "you still turn me on" message.

Consequently, scenes between partners have risks that scenes between strangers don't have. Hitting rough spots with a partner usually hurts more than with a stranger (which can be plenty bad enough). One of the scariest moments in any relationship is that first time we wonder if the sexual part might be slipping away forever. Ironically, for some, the fear of the thing can make the thing itself happen. Put simply, fear of failure is a "soft on."

There are many ways by which the playing together part of the relationship⁻ gets into trouble. Partners who pressure themselves to have a successful scene stop being able to be spontaneous with their sexuality. This fear is commonly known as "performance anxiety."

Bottoms can worry that they are not heavy enough or that the Top will stumble across the one play activity where their true wimpiness will be revealed at last. Tops can worry about the need they may feel to produce constantly escalating scenes, or that they are approaching the edge of their technical competence. If a Top has made a serious technical error in a scene recently, he may be feeling "gun shy" about playing for a while. These are just a few examples to give you the idea—opportunities for developing performance anxiety are infinite.

When anybody in the relationship has performance anxiety, there will often be subtle attempts to sabotage making a scene happen. One or the other might pick a fight on "play" night so as to make himself unattractive. Or he might develop a headache, or hurt himself in the garden, or ruin dinner—the list of possible ploys is endless, but the objective is to carefully obstruct movement toward a scene. Most often, this is all unconscious, but sometimes he knows just what he is up to, and is powerless to stop himself. Both Tops and bottoms do it.

These are good times to talk: "I'm not feeling much like a scene tonight because ...I look fat and feel unattractive, or I watched you cruising today, and I am worried that maybe you are getting tired of me, or Your mother is coming to visit, and that pisses me off, or I am afraid you will want to do such and such to me, and it scares me." Whatever, but tell the truth, or at least as much truth as you can stand.

This gets the feelings about the relationship out in the open where they can be dealt with. It is usually much harder for most men to get into a scene when there is unfinished relationship business lying around all over the place. I am not saying that playing at such times is impossible, but the scenes may feel flatter, or just like mere technical exercises rather than flights of ecstasy for both.

Work with my clients has taught me that the worst times to play with your partner(s) are when anyone is angry or depressed. SM can be wonderful stuff, but it does not have the power to cure these ailments anymore than love conquers all.

Men who decide to play rather than talk about problems cannot be surprised if the scene is not wonderful. SM was never designed to carry the burden of solving relationship problems. Men who try to make it do so will come away feeling that SM has let them down in some way. This will make it even harder to play the next time.

How sex works physiologically is not much of a mystery any more. How it works psychologically is now partly known, but mostly not. The psychology of an SM scene *as it is unfolding* has never been studied to my knowledge. What I have learned about it comes from extending information about sexuality in general into the realm of SM, and from many long conversations with sadomasochists both in and out of the therapy room.

One of the concepts from sexuality research that I think men in SM relationships will be able to make much good use of is "cuing." The idea is that we constantly send each other signals about what we want and what we don't want. Cues may be verbal (with words), visual (movements), or sonic (with sounds). Some Tops may not know it, but one reason for using a blindfold is to eliminate visual cues and focus the bottom on touch or sound.

Cues inform without actually having to make a speech or draw a diagram. This cuing thing is something that we *all* do all the time when we are with others. It is very subtle, but with conscious effort, anyone can learn more about it, and improve his cuing skills. In general, the sexual parts of relationships tend to be most satisfying when the giving and receiving of cues is smoothly worked out, so this stuff is important.

Not all cuing has sexual purposes. When we are hungry, we may signal the fact by rubbing our stomach and appearing to be in discomfort. Our hope is that the person for whom the cue is intended will say something like, "Are you hungry yet?" Another example: A quick glance toward the sky with an exasperated look is the nonverbal way of saying, "Gimme a break."

To make this idea concrete for you, let's think about some common cues that Tops and bottoms exchange. When bottoms cruise boots in a way that is sure to be noticed by the wearer, that is a cue. The cue says, "I want closer contact with your boots, Mister." It is a more powerful erotic signal than simply reporting to someone you think is hot that "one thing I like is boots."

My belief about successful playing is that Tops and bottoms relay to each other, in rapid-fire succession, cues which are loaded with information about preferences, taste in stimulation, intentions and responses to various stimulations.

In a way, a scene is a mutual feedback loop in which the bottom's response to a Top's stimulations becomes the next cue to the Top about where to go next. A bottom's reaction to the stroke of a whip will influence (but not necessarily control) the Top's next stroke (if the Top is responsive, that is.)

When bottoms refuse to react to anything, Tops are forced to draw their own conclusions about just where the bottom is at. Without reactions (one type of cue), Tops are generally playing in the dark so to speak, because there are no cues to read. This is partly why Tops complain about what I call "grin-and-bear-it-bottoms."

When you are horny and want to get into a scene, you must cue your partner as to your readiness to play. He cannot read your mind after all. If you think about it, that is what we do when we cruise in bars and other places—we find ways to code our readiness to get it on. If we determine through cuing that the interest is mutual, then we move toward negotiations. If the negotiations are successful, a scene happens, either right then or later.

We often assume that once partnered, the need to cruise is over. Not true. The content of the cruising changes, meaning we must start using different cues. In a bar, you might stare at a stranger to signal your interest. If you did that in a relationship, he would ask if anything was wrong. The meaning of the cue has been changed by the context.

In a relationship you might sit at his feet after dinner to send the same message. Tops might just decide that it is a good time to saddle soap their favorite whip, or send for their leather.

Some partnerships have worked out very explicit and detailed cuing that helps them move into playing. One might shower after dinner to signal interest. Or put on special music. Or offer to bring a drink. Or ask, "Would you like it if I polished your boots now?" The list of possibilities is endless. Be creative.

One way to cue your partner is to take your suit off when you get home and go naked in boots or maybe a favorite jock or the vest you like—he will get your message if he wants to. If not, you still get to be in your favorite things anyway. It does not take two to be sexy. You found each other sexy before you were together, didn't you?

In relationships it is easy to forget that everyone likes to be seduced. One advantage to being in a relationship is that we don't have to start from ignorance every time we play. Good SM takes practice. In relationships, we learn how to turn our partners on. We know what works and what doesn't. All of this is not an excuse to skip the seduction part of having a scene. If you want to keep things hot, remember to turn each other on when you are horny.

Moving toward a scene will be more successful if you keep two things in mind: first, work hard and often to keep the unfinished emotional business in the relationship to a minimum. Second, remember that when you are sexy and seductive (whatever that means to you) you will get to play more often. Learn what cues work and use them.

Smoothing Out The Rough Spots

All relationships have difficulties, and those couples who share an interest in SM are no exception. Yet quite often, when dominance and submission are part of a couple's sexual style, there can be special difficulties that come up when they attempt to solve their problems. Since most kinky couples have no role models to be guided by, they will often do their level best to work things out for themselves with whatever skills they may have. Typically, they don't turn up in the therapy room until they have come to a serious impasse and they both decide that they need professional help to get through the difficulty.

But because kinky couples are usually so reluctant to discuss the sexual aspects of their relationship, they will often delay professional support until well past the point where a professional could have been of assistance. This is like the medical patient who so fears doctors that he waits until he is at death's door before seeking treatment. When this happens, the illness may have already done so much damage to the body that treatment comes too late to save the patient's life or limb. When it comes to a couple's private life together, this fear of professional helpers can itself be responsible for letting the relationship deteriorate past the point of no return. So, the relationship disintegrates. The partners decide it is just easier to break up and try again with someone else, maybe. Whenever I have come across such a situation, I find myself wishing that they had come to seek help with problem solving sooner. All therapists are sad to see people who love each other fail at "marriage" when that was what they had originally wanted and tried for.

Although it is impossible to detail all the sorts of problems that can break relationships apart, I think it is safe to offer one guideline that can be helpful in preventing unnecessary divorce when used early enough. It is probably most important for the individual who notices it first to be honest with himself about the fact that he feels what I will call "persistent emotional pain" that doesn't feel good. There is no telling which partner might feel it first; it can be the Top or the bottom, but it is very important not to pretend that he doesn't feel it at all, or that it doesn't really matter.

Most commonly, this persistent emotional pain will appear as a depression, a sadness that won't go away. The pain can also sometimes masquerade as a simmering anger or resentment. Most people will often feel this way for a while before they even notice it. One day you just realize that you've been really down in the dumps for weeks or that your temper has been really short for a good while.

Sometimes the persistent emotional pain won't really come to your attention until you suddenly realize that your behavior has really changed in some important way recently. Maybe you have been drinking (or drugging) a lot more, or a lot more often lately. Maybe you notice that you have started drinking at home (or at bars) much more often than was your habit. Maybe you don't initiate sex much or maybe you get "headaches" when sex comes up whereas, before, you were eager for it. Maybe you've been hitting the junk food trail, and have suddenly gained 15 unwanted pounds. Maybe you are suddenly missing a lot of work or skipping class more than is usual for you. Whatever the change, any of these sorts of things can be a signal that might help you identify a persistent emotional pain.

However you discover it, the very first thing to do once you realize you feel this way, is to share this fact with your partner. It is not necessary to "figure out the reason" for the pain before you notify your partner about it, just report it. And right here is the place where being in a dominant/submissive relationship can really get in the way. Tops can take the attitude that it is not okay to let a bottom know that something is wrong emotionally because he may fear that his bottom will lose respect for him or think him weak or un-masculine in some way. A bottom can take the attitude that his Top/Master has more important things on his mind, and won't want to be bothered. Or, a bottom might also decide that his feelings are weak or un-masculine. Most of us are brought up believing that "real men" don't admit to feeling emotional pain. Well, that is bull shit, folks. Anyone can feel this kind of emotional pain, and you ignore it at your own peril, *and* at the peril of the relationship. Failure to deal with unexpressed emotional pain early on is probably the most common reason for relationship failure.

Sharing your awareness of this pain can take many forms depending on your own style. It might sound like this, for example, "I'm in a bad way lately, and I don't yet know just why or what it's all about, but I thought you should know." Or maybe, "I just realized that I've been snapping at you a lot lately, and I just *got* that I'm hurting inside over something. I don't know what, and I think maybe that's why I've been so bitchy." Or even, "Something is wrong with me lately, and it has me worried." Although saying it out loud is the better way, some of you may find that doing it in a note or a letter is the only way that feels right. Whether you speak the words or write them, try to say as much as you know about the feelings, but don't try to have things all figured out before you start the process. This way, you involve your partner in the problem solving right from the start which helps him feel more a part of your life—your whole life, not just the parts that he can see.

Try to choose a good time for delivering this information about yourself. Don't just drop this information on him, then run out the door for work or hop on an airplane for a week-long business trip. Don't hit him with this news when he is home from work with a bad cold, or whenever he is likely to be distracted and unable to pay full attention to you. Don't do it when you are with others or have been drinking all night, right before or after sex, just before you have house guests arriving to stay for a week, and so on. Choose a moment when there will be enough time to provide any details you may have about the feelings, and allow at least an hour for possible conversation.

Once you have shared the information, take time to talk

with him about what your thoughts are about the pain every time you find a new piece of the puzzle for yourself. Keep him updated. When you even suspect that he may have a role in your feeling, for God's sake, tell him what you think *might* be going on. Then listen to his thoughts about it. Try to make statements about yourself: "When you do such and such, I start to feel so and so."

Sometimes, there is no "good time" to share your new awareness about this feeling. If he was just laid off from work and is worried about finding a new job, or just found out he was HIV positive, or that a parent or friend has just died, then you are justified in waiting maybe a week or so before you decide to share the news until he has had a chance to adjust a bit to changes in his own life. But even when yours is just another piece of bad or difficult news in his life, it is still important to tell it like it is. Part of being a couple means facing life—its joys *and* its troubles—together, as a team. When one person in a relationship has a problem, both have that same problem whether the other one knows about the difficulty or not.

Once you both know that one of you is suffering from a persistent emotional pain, there are two problem solvers available to tackle the issues instead of just one. The ability to work on issues together successfully is one of the things that confirms two people as a couple. If you are going to keep important personal matters a secret, then what is the point of being in a relationship in the first place. Being "lovers" or "married" is not just about sharing the good stuff. It must include involving your partner in your life as it really is.

Fear that you are a "bad" partner for sharing such information, or that your man will reject you unless you are always "just fine" will not help you here. Furthermore, any guy who tries to make you feel bad for having such feelings is just a fair-weather lover and not worth your affections. Once we decide we really want a relationship, we all need to be involved with men who are willing to participate *fully* in our inner life—our emotional life—as well as our external lives. A relationship must be a safe place in which to feel all the feelings that go with being alive and in the world. Otherwise, why bother?

Just because two people can fall in love and choose to be together is no guarantee that the guy we pick is willing to go through the emotional tough spots with us. Check this out during the dating process to see if he can really hang in there when you are going through your own growing pains. Don't overlook this important piece of information about a man you date just because he is good sex. You will be facing problems together long after you have settled into a comfortable sexuality together.

Part Two

THE COMMUNITY
COMMENTARIES

Editor's Note On
The Community Commentaries

Guy Baldwin places tremendous importance on the relationships people have with one another as families, communities, and interacting segments of the overall social network. It is only natural that he would, being a psychotherapist. Or, perhaps more aptly, it is only natural that a man with his deep concern for such relationships would become a psychotherapist. The same interest in relationships, particularly on the scale of communities, was evidenced earlier when, in 1971, Baldwin finished his undergraduate studies at the University of Colorado with a major in Anthropology.

In any case, it is this long-standing and deeply-felt concern that underpins the essays in this section. What informs the content of these essays, and elevates Baldwin's thoughts to a potentially prescriptive state, is that he has lived and succeeded in the leather community for more than two decades. And, increasingly over the past many years, he has taken a position of leadership within the emerging national leather communities.

I have been guided in the arrangement and editing of this section primarily by Baldwin's own suggestions. The sequence and style work wonders in expressing a positive mood about the history and possibilities of leatherfolk in groups.

Glass Houses

"All the world is but a mirror...look if you dare!"

—The Aspirant Sage

For generations, elements in Western society have said that homosexuals are perverts because we commit "unnatural acts." This "unnatural acts" stuff has often been used to justify the hatred that so many people feel toward gay men, lesbians and the sexually different—like, say, for example us leather/SM folks.

The message about unnatural acts comes at us from parents, teachers, religious and political leaders, kids on the street, movie characters—everywhere. For as long as I can remember, my instant reaction to these messages was usually a kind of frightened and defensive anger. I didn't stop to think about it; I just got mad. I guess I got mad because I knew they were wrong. For me, being homosexual is natural. There is nothing in me that I must fight with in order to be attracted to another man (assuming that he turns me on, of course). Homosexuality is my nature.

One reason that our detractors get upset with our differentness is that because homosexuality is not natural *for them*, they assume that it can't be natural for anyone else. Since heterosexuality is so natural *for them*, they conclude that it is the natural state for us, too. They point to their greater numbers to justify their conclusion.

Unfortunately, mainstream gays and lesbians use essentially the same justification to put down those of us who also happen to be into SM/leather/fetish sexualities. Our sexuality and love making doesn't look like their gay sexuality, so they conclude that there must be something wrong with it. Again, there are messages about how unnatural we are. Yet, once again, nothing could be and feel more natural *for me*.

Recently, I have begun to think more carefully about this word, unnatural. It means, "not found in nature," or perhaps, "not of nature." Well, even an untrained observer can look at nature, and notice lots of things that turn out to be very damned important to all us so called perverts.

Look into the heavens and you will find that there are many sorts of stars out there, not just one kind. Likewise, there are many different kinds of planets in our own solar system—no two are really alike.

Here on Earth, there are many ways to be a tree, or a rock, or a horse. The consistent message we get from nature is diversity and variety—many kinds of ants, many kinds of spider webs. Watch wildlife documentaries for a year and you will discover that there is great variation in animal behavior too.

There are lots of ways for adult animals to care for their young—sometimes it is the male that guards them, and sometimes not. There is also great diversity in mating behavior among animals. Animals don't all fuck the same way; just watch National Geographic and you will learn all this and more.

Something else that you will learn is that all this variety fits together very nicely and neatly onto something called Earth. Each animal, no matter how strange and unexpected the behavior might seem, plays its part in the great scheme of nature. There seems to be a place for all this great diversity, and it somehow all works together. Variety and diversity are nature's theme song. Look around you. It is everywhere, this diversity.

When we apply this rule of nature to ourselves, we quickly discover that there must also be many ways to be a man, many ways to be a woman, various ways to be sexual, and lots of ways to make love. We already know this, why can't the religious and political conservatives get it?

This means that the real perverts and perpetrators of unnatural acts are those individuals (preachers, politicians, spokespersons for citrus industries, disco divas, and comics)

102

who think that our sex life ought to look just like theirs.

The truly unnatural thing is for our supposedly American institutions (church, family, school, law, medicine) to suppress or reduce human diversity and variety to make us all look and behave alike. Humans are not simply interchangeable parts designed to fit smoothly into a well-oiled society like disposable spark plugs.

The really unnatural act is to oppose variety and diversity. It is anti-nature to force people into what appears to be the common mold just because it is common. We all know that "common" does not necessarily mean "better."

Leather/SM/fetish sexuality is obviously a natural part of human sexual diversity. As such, it is a perfect reflection of nature both on Earth and in the Cosmos.

We Do It Too!

Twenty two years ago when I was just coming out into the leather/SM scene, the first thing I noticed was how alike most of the men in the bar looked. The second thing that caught my attention was how many rules there seemed to be: don't mix brown and black leather; don't mix brass trim with silver trim; never be seen wearing anything but boots in public; bike caps are for Tops, bottoms go with heads bare; wear a (black) belt or don't go around the Men Who Do—and many, many others.

Not knowing any better, I conformed and promptly became one of the more militant enforcers of these rules myself. After all, we had to have ways of telling who was real and who was phony. Just like the Shriners, the Mummers, the Boy Scouts and the Los Angeles Fire Department, we had to know who belonged and who did not by looking at the uniform. Unfortunately all this made it possible to wear leather only on your body—it was not necessary to have it in your heart.

Anyhow, there was one set of rules for us insiders to follow so that we could feel closer, I guess. But there was a second set of rules about how to deal with outsiders: don't explain who We are or what We do; always make snide remarks about drag

103

queens and those who are feminine in any way (just like homophobic straights); distrust those who look or act differently than We look and act (just like homophobic straights). We were, or thought We were, the elite. We "accidentally" burned sweaters with cigarettes in the Ramrod and the Toolbox whenever the tourists came in to gawk at us. I saw it; I laughed about it; I did it myself.

And, as a group, we fashioned a separate world for ourselves that was far from the gay mainstream. There was always some occasional crossover into the Land of Vanilla, but we didn't admit to it much. Leather life became ex-clusive, not in-clusive. We helped create the gulf that exists between us and the mainstream community in just this way—with our arrogant tightness.

It took me an embarrassingly long time (it takes what it takes, I suppose) to recognize the awful similarity between the rigidity among leathermen and, say, the rigidity of the nuns I grew to hate and fear as a boy—same tightness of spirit, different habit, but same color—or the similarity between Old Guard leathermen and the religious, political and social personalities who also oppose diversity and variety.

None of this is meant to ignore all the good things that early leathermen did accomplish, such as the very first organized fund raising with which gay men helped each other financially. In many clubs, bike club brothers helped with medical expenses when one of their own had a bike accident or some other personal disaster strike.

Nevertheless, we were one very intolerant (scared?) bunch of guys. We were intolerant of variety among leather men and we were quick to discourage too much experimentation, especially in appearance. And we were especially intolerant of anything that smacked of femininity.

Gentlemen, it is unlikely that we will ever win the war for tolerance of our lifestyle against the powerful forces who wish to press us into a straight and vanilla mold until we are first willing to tolerate the variety that exists among our own kind.

Much of this variety and diversity occurs among the

104

younger guys just coming into the scene. Our community is in danger of losing a generation of younger newcomers unless we are willing to loosen up and allow what is in their nuts to dictate how they dress and act. For many of them, the military influences so prevalent when I was young are often missing entirely in their erotic life. And there are many who just don't relate to the stiff semi-military look that has been common in leather bars for so long.

Younger newcomers to the leather scene may have different ideas about what is sexy than we had 20 years ago. We knew Marlon Brando and James Dean, lots of soldiers and lots of cops; they know Mel Gibson and Tom Cruise. We had Flash Gordon and the Lone Ranger, and they have Luke Skywalker, Axl Rose, Billy Idol and Sting. It is reasonable for these newcomers to leather/SM/fetish sexuality to want to dress and act in a way that is "hot" for them (now called "cool" by the way).

And, it is okay for us old timers not to get turned on by it. Just 'cause it doesn't make your dick hard doesn't mean you have to be impolite or hostile, or not tell them how to handle a whip or use rope if they ask. It seems a shame to let all that knowledge we have acquired go nowhere just because the person asking for it has a mohawk haircut.

Welcome these frontiersmen as you, yourself would wish to be welcomed. Do unto others...

"Old Guard": Its Origins, Traditions, Mystique and Rules

While reading an interview of Brian Dawson, one of the leather community's better-known leaders, I came across some of his comments about the "Old Guard" in the leather lifestyle. Although I used that label in a piece I wrote almost three years ago, I only recently realized that there was a strong likelihood that large numbers of leather guys don't quite know for sure what the phrase "Old Guard" really means. I'm sure I have never seen a description of the style (and it is a style), so I want to offer one now. I have carried my own "Old Guard" card in my wallet right next to my Selective Service Registration card (draft card) for long enough that I probably qualify to offer what follows.

First, a bit of historical perspective will be more helpful than you might guess. "Old Guard" is really a misnomer—a misapplied name—for the earliest set of habits that jelled by the mid-to late 1950s in the men's leather community here in the U.S. It is very important to remember that the modern leather scene as we now know it first formalized itself out of the group of men who were soldiers returning home after World War II (1939-1945).

For many gay men of that era, their World War II military service was their first homosocial experience (first time being thrown together mostly in the company of other men for significant lengths of time), their first time away from their growing-up places, and their first experience of male bonding during periods of high stress. War was (and is) serious business. People died, buddies depended on each other for their lives, and the chips were down. Discipline was the order of the day, and

107

the nation believed that only discipline and dedication would win the war and champion freedom. (Ever notice the especially strong patriotic feelings that happen at leather events?)

Anyway, these gay war veterans learned about the value and pleasure of discipline and hard work in the achievement of a noble purpose. They also learned how to play hard when they got the chance for leave time. Indeed, military life during wartime was (and is) a mix of emotional extremes born out of sure knowledge that one could literally be "here today, and gone tomorrow." Lastly (for these purposes), the gay vets had the secret knowledge that they fought and served every bit as well as straight soldiers, and this information strengthened their self-esteem. All of these things came to be associated with the disciplined, military way of life as it existed during the wartime years.

Although not all gay men of that time served in the military, those who didn't were exposed to the military attitudes through their contact with the vast numbers of military men who were everywhere to be seen and cruised both during and immediately after the war years. In any case, all these things greatly influenced the shape of masculine gay sexualities.

Upon their return to the States, about 1946, many of the gay vets wanted to retain the most satisfying elements of their military experience and at the same time, hang out socially and sexually with other masculine gay men. They found that only in the swashbuckling motorcycle culture did such opportunities exist, so gay bike clubs were born. It was here that they found the combination of easy camaraderie, the stress and thrill of real risk taking (the riding), and the masculine sexuality that they had known during their military days.

Since one can tell who is and is not in the military only when uniforms are worn, these gay men unconsciously (in most cases) transferred their loyalties to their own uniform—the leather gear of bike riders with a few paramilitary touches thrown in. Club insignia often recalled the insignia of special military units: Thunderbolts, Warriors, Blue Max, and Iron Cross to name only a few. Club members would exchange their insignia with members of other clubs in friendship. Christening rituals were transferred from tanks, ships and airplanes to motorcycles, and piss was substituted for champagne. The military dress uniform hats became the leather bike caps. All these elements were representative of things just as they had been during military service.

Incidentally, during the war, the soldiers would often put on skits for their own amusement. Since women were not allowed at the front, some of the men would play the parts of women by doing a kind of mock dress-up (as in one scene from "South Pacific"). Later, this tradition would be expressed in "drag" shows during bike runs. So, masculine men pretended to be pretending to be women—not truly "drag" at all. (It still happens in a few places.)

In any case, being in the military also meant following lots of rules. And, just as in the military, there were (unspoken) rules about what you did and did not wear, how you handled your personal affairs, who you could and could not socialize with, and more. All this was overlaid with a kind of ritual formalism just as in the military. Those men who were really into dominance and submission, SM, or leather sex tended to take these rules rather more seriously than those guys who simply thought of themselves as butch. The butch ones wore just enough leather to be practical when riding, and those into the exotic sexualities tended to wear more gear than necessary to signal this fact about themselves, but they all hung out together in the same settings. As you might guess, in some cases, any particular person might be into both riding *and* the exotic sexualities.

Just as an aside here, before and during the war, kinky folks seeking to identify each other would sometimes defensively ask, "Do you play the mandolin or the saxophone?" to discover which of them was the masochist or the sadist by the first letter of these instruments. All this while wearing street clothes! The creation of a butch subculture by the gay vets began to allow people to specialize their sexual interests in a way that had been impossible earlier. Prior to this development, it was not

109

apparent that there were very many ways to be gay.

The bike clubs and the bars where they hung out became the magnets of their day which attracted those gay men who were interested in the masculine end of the gay spectrum, but is was the leather men who defined the masculine extreme at that time. (Nowadays, we know that there are many ways to be masculine.)

This meant that those who had an inclination to kinky action pretty much felt compelled to explore kink in the context of the leather/SM scene since it was the only game in town. If motorcycle riding or black leather itself was not "your thing," you still felt obligated to visit the hangouts, and look and act the part as much as possible. There was no other way to get access to the inner circle of those who looked like they knew something about the exotic sexualities. This meant finding out what the rules of *inclusion* were (how can I be included?). To some extent, all this is still true because the attitude still prevails that the "uniform" indicates experience and social access to the Knowledgeable People.

And so, the scene became ex-clusive rather than in-clusive, meaning that the people in the scene understood the rules and tried to keep outsiders out—to exclude them. An outsider became defined as anyone (butch or not) who did not have a primary interest in and experience with the exotic sexualities, or at least an interest in motorcycles. (This excluding attitude was probably also reinforced by guilt about being kinky.)

I know that this combination of kinky men mixed in with motorcycle riders may sound a bit odd now, but that's how the scene worked and, to some slight extent, still does. All through the 80's, with the emergence of kinky organizations and specifically leather/SM events, the motorcycle riding community and the kinky/leather community have grown apart such that now those in one group are pretty much ignorant of or indifferent to the events happening in the other. This growing separation is more true in larger cities which have the numbers of people necessary to separately support the needs and agendas of these two communities. Consequently, many old and venerable bike clubs have experienced a drop in membership and some have disbanded altogether.

But for the most part, kinky people have segregated themselves out from the riders as the process of erotic specialization has continued. Generally, the riding community seems not to have minded this development, perhaps because many of the members of riding clubs are either turned off or embarrassed by the erotic visibility of the kinky crowd. Birds of a feather...

But for this discussion, it is noteworthy that many of those kinky people *retained* the paramilitary trappings, manners and attitudes of that early, core group of returning World War II gay vets. Most importantly, these features of the military mind-set joined with kinky interests and became erotic in and of themselves—became fetishes. These men then, were the original "Old Guard," and so it will come as no surprise that their quasi-military rules of inclusion and exclusion still influence kinky society today.

So, what exactly were the (unspoken) "Old Guard" rules? Here are a few of the more important ones that had come into force by 1970.

About Attire: Always wear boots, butch ones, and preferably black. Always wear a wide black leather belt—plain, not fancy. Never mix brown leather with black leather. Never mix chrome or silver trim with gold or brass trim. Long pants only, Levis or leather, and no shorts. Chaps indicate more commitment than levis, and leather pants more commitment than chaps, especially when worn consistently. Leather jackets must have epaulets (bike riders excepted). Head gear is reserved for Tops or experienced or heavy bottoms only.

Bottoms may not own collars unless a particular Top has allowed that bottom to be the custodian of the Top's collar. A bottom wearing a collar is a slave, and belongs to the owner of the collar who, presumably, has the keys. Other Tops are not to engage a collared bottom in conversation, but other bottoms may do so. Should such a relationship end, the collar must be returned to the Top.

Never touch the bill of a bike cap, including your own. Never touch another man's cap (or head gear) unless you are very intimate friends or lovers.

Keep studs and other decorations to a tasteful minimum unless they happen to be club insignia. Never wear another man's leather unless he puts it on you. Leather other than boots and belt must be "earned" through the achievement of successively challenging scenes. Wearing gloves is reserved for heavy players, glove fetishists or bike riders.

Always indicate SM preference, only with keys left for Top, or right for bottom. If you are cruising seriously, wear the keys out; if not seriously, tuck them in a back pocket. Always indicate strictly leather sex or "rough sex" interest by wearing no keys at all. Those who "switch" are second class players and not to be taken as seriously because they haven't made their minds up. If you must switch, do so in another town.

"Full" leather is reserved for after 10:00 P.M. only and only with "our own kind." Respect the public by wearing less of it during the day. Don't frighten old ladies (I did once by accident), or anyone else for that matter.

About Socializing & Cruising: Experience in the scene determines social seniority (Top or bottom), not age, not size, not amount of leather worn, and not offices held in organizations, awards received or titles won.

Tops and experienced bottoms should be accorded higher respect and deference *unless* and *until* they behave rudely—all are expected to observe rules of social courtesy—bad manners are inexcusable and can lower one's status in the scene (thereby reducing access to the Knowledgeable People for information or play).

Real leathermen keep their word. They do not borrow or lend money. They conduct their affairs with honor and integrity. They don't lie.

Preliminary social contact should be on the formal side. "Senior Persons" (Top or bottom) are not to be interrupted when in conversation. Experience being *equal*, Tops lead the conversation, Junior Tops defer to Senior Tops and Senior

112

bottoms in social situations. Junior bottoms defer to all others in the scene but not to outsiders.

When walking together, bottoms walk half-a-step behind and to the left of Tops with whom they are involved or playing.

It is up to the Top or the experienced bottom to extend a hand to invite a handshake. (All touching is highly restricted during initial contact between strangers.)

Never over-indulge in drugs or alcohol in public, or otherwise attract scornful attention to one's self—to do so brings dishonor on the men in the scene.

Tops should always have the first two opportunities to make verbal or physical contact. The more submissive one is, the less direct eye contact one makes—glance frequently at or stare at a man's boots *only* when cruising, less so in non-sexual conversation. The more dominant one is, the more direct the eye contact is unless there is no erotic interest (cruising only).

Men in the scene do not discuss (or write about!) the scene with outsiders. All men in the scene must be able to spot outsiders with the "right stuff," and be ready to facilitate them into the scene after they indicate *sincere* interest.

General Rules: None of these rules are taught or explained to anyone except by innuendo, inference, or example. Erotic technical information is only shared among peers. Maintain formal and non-committal relationships with those outside the scene; avoid contact with feminine men. Women are not allowed, although Senior People may occasionally have intellectual or brief social relationships with a qualified kinky woman, but only rarely and only in private.

Very few men maintained full compliance with all these rules all the time, and some flatly refused to follow rules they personally objected to. But, to be included, one was expected to follow at least most of these rules most of the time. Also, confusingly, there was some variation in some of the rules depending on what city you happened to be in at the time. The list above is not complete although it conveys the sense of the style.

Understandably, a certain stiffness surrounded the men who

followed these rules, just as a certain stiffness surrounded the military men of the era. Those who sought inclusion had the challenge of finding a relaxed and easy-going way to follow the rules. However, this required considerable social skill and many kinky people lacking those skills (or patience) simply gave up and accepted a frustrated role on the fringe.

As time passed, there were more and more guys in their twenties whose early sexual development had *not* been influenced strongly by contact with the military. Therefore, they lacked the early raw material with which to fetishize the military features of the Old Guard leather/SM scene. Still, they needed information and experiences to help shape the urges of insistent kinky longings.

These people were essentially without resources until the establishment of relatively recent kinky organizations that have created educational opportunities *not* bound by Old Guard rules. Consequently, there is a lot more support now for new people coming into the leather/SM scene who have other ideas (non-military) about what is hot. Long hair, rockers with wild designs on their jackets, road racing bikers with brightly colored leathers, leather faeries, skinheads, women and others now are found on turf that was once dominated by the "Old Guard" system.

So, what I and others have called the Old Guard should perhaps be thought of as "Early Guard" or maybe "First Guard," because that style makes sense given the erotic influences that shaped the inner lives of the men who were coming of age sexually at that time. The Old Guard made some real contributions and made some real mistakes, and still does both. It is more useful to understand than to criticize. And, perhaps most importantly, what the Old Guard did for the development and expansion of kinky life and butch gay male sexuality can best be appreciated against the backdrop of what had existed earlier—not much of anything!

But remember this, as long as we have a military, and a paramilitary police system, and as long as that military has traditions of initiation, ritual, inclusion/exclusion, honor and service, there will always be an "Old Guard." Its size and influence in the leather/SM scene will probably always be proportional to the role played by the military and other paramilitary organizations in society—larger following wartime and smaller during peace.

I thought maybe you'd like to know.

Teach Them A Little Bit

*"Sometimes doing the right thing is hard, and
doing the wrong thing is easy. This is the ground
where integrity grows. It is often a
demanding crop to harvest."*

—The Aspirant Sage

Many of us have vanilla friends and/or family—yes, lovers
too—who discover in one way or another that we pursue a
leather/SM lifestyle. Some of these people will bring themselves
to ask us questions about our sexuality. These can be tense
moments.

It is not easy to refuse a true friend information that might
bring us still closer. Yet we also fear that the truth might stress
the friendship past its breaking point. The only way I know of
to avoid this situation completely is just not to allow ourselves
to become close to non-kinky people. That's hard.

Each of us makes a sometimes difficult decision about
whether to explain, just how much to explain, what to explain,
and how to go about explaining something so diverse and
complex as the leather/SM scene. Clearly, the easiest thing is to
sidestep the issue with a sly diversion, a denial, a deception of
some sort. Or is it?

Vanilla folks will continue to think of us as sexual outlaws,
as real and dangerous perverts, unless we can somehow give
them information that might help their view of us to change.
Our pornography is already under attack by the anti-violence
people and Postal authorities. There is lots of evidence that we
are losing ground.

Just as with the gay movement, society mostly changes its
view "one person at a time" so to speak. By this, I mean that
the cutting edge of social change is one real person explaining

117

himself or herself to one other real person.

I am a person who wants to help make the world a safe place for kinky folk of all kinds. Furthermore, I have discovered that I can soften bigots and turn some of them into supporters with friendly education. For me, it is a bit like talking a nervous bottom through a scene that he is afraid of.

My vanilla buddies used to think all SM/leather sex was another version of applied homophobia. Now, they know that only occasionally is SM used in such destructive ways—that much more often, people feel great about what they do in a scene. I have taken the time to chip away at their prejudice, and bit by bit, they have become allowing and tolerant. And, they are all registered to vote!

I know that the Old Guard position on this dictates that "the less they know about us the better." That may have been true at one time, but now they know a little bit, and "only a little knowledge" is dangerous.

There are elements in religious, political and police leadership who have just enough information about us to provoke their worst fears. The Meese commission was not a paranoid fantasy, it really happened and has real consequences for us. We have already become too visible to slide, unnoticed, back into our corner of the world to quietly pursue our brand of ecstacy.

For all these reasons our relationships with vanilla folks take on a new importance. As a group, kinky people need vanilla friends. One day we may need them to defend us, perhaps in ways we cannot yet even imagine. Remember that it is never just gay folks who defeat anti-gay legislation. Repeatedly, laws against us would pass without lots of help from informed heterosexuals. The same necessities exist for kinky people. Besides, it will be better to have more vanilla people on our side and not need them, than to need them and not have them.

Giving your vanilla friends, family and lovers a friendly and *appropriate* education about your lifestyle will help make a more tolerant world for us all. How to do it? What are the issues?

1) Spend some quiet, private time with yourself first. Use this time to think about and maybe write down your own answers to questions that you think (hope?) (fear?) you might be asked someday. Speak the questions out loud and make your answers out loud while you visualize the person right in front of you. Look into their eyes.

2) Before you answer real questions from real people, assess the intelligence, age, and experience of the person asking and try to make your answer fit all three when possible. Speak in the same type of language that your listener uses.

3) Before you answer, find out why they are asking. Some of the people who like us are also not very nice as individuals. They may be searching for a way to hurt or belittle somehow. I strongly suggest that you do not even try to answer if you sense that there is an unkind motive. When I sense unkindness, I always say so, and it puts them on the defensive when it's true.

4) Keep your answers short, interesting and witty at first if possible. This tends to lead them more deeply into the subject. Talk in generalities early in the conversation and specifics later on, if at all. *Retain your privacy*—you don't have to "tell all." You can make informative remarks about the scene without telling others how you participate in it. Would they tell you the intimate details of their sex life, including their fantasies? Would you want to know?

5) Watch for reactions to what you are saying. Read their faces. If you detect that you have just said something that made them uncomfortable, stop. Then remark that such and such seems to have made them uncomfortable, and explain your point in more detail (or less detail) until your listener is comfortable again. Then proceed if you think they are ready to hear more. If they are not ready, then "thus endeth the lesson." Don't tell people more than they want to know. It turns off their curiosity about the subject.

6) You don't have to explain it all at once. Say a little to make them keep asking questions. That way, they must accept

responsibility for their education. When you think you have answered their questions, ask them if they feel their question has been answered. If they think not, say more. Offer help with future questions.

7) We are not sexual anarchists, but vanilla folks think so. Correct this impression by stressing the principals of safe, sane and consensual. Loosely, safe means that care is taken to prevent accidental physical or psychological injury and that procedures are followed that prevent the transmission of disease. Sane means that those who play together are mentally in charge of themselves, and that they are also not under undue influence of drugs, including alcohol. Consensual means that any player has the ability to influence the pace and intensity of an encounter and may end it at will.

8) If you don't know something, say so. It is dangerous to pretend that you know more than you really do know. It places you in a position to misinform, and that is not your purpose. The objective is to support their interest in you and your life in a friendly way.

9) Keep your hostility out of the conversation. It turns people off to what you have to say. Themes of sexual variation and personal erotic freedom do better than hurt and anger to get and keep their attention.

10) Just as when good parents answer those first questions from their children about sex and babies, so too must we be careful to explain without apology, for that is partly what creates the impression of guilt. And we do not need to feel guilt about what we do so long as we harness these energies for the purposes of creating good times and good feelings with each other, and not destruction.

11) Perhaps most importantly, try to find something else in their life that they know well and describe the scene in terms that are familiar to them.

Here's an example. One of my favorite ways of talking to outsiders about the scene is to liken it to a cafeteria. When we are horny, it is like being hungry at the beginning of a cafeteria or smorgasbord line, standing there with our empty plate. We do kind of the same thing when we want to play. We put together whatever sexual "meal" suits our fancy at the time. There are many kinds of "dishes" offered by the scene, and no one is expected to like or try all that is available. I never met anyone who likes it all.

There are "platters" labeled, whips, condom fucking, bondage, pain, fisting (gloves, of course), master/slave stuff, blood, jackoff, piss, shit, kissing, rubber, leather, tit trips, cowboy, indian, needles, gags, verbal scenes, cross dressing, catheters, dildoes, electricity, vomit, outdoors, indoors, temperature scenes, and on and on. In any combination.

Usually, I will change the list of things I mention depending on the person I am talking to. I then go on to say that the list also includes whipped cream, feathers, chocolate syrup, whiskers, ice cream, fresh strawberries, marshmallows, warm baby oil, lace, fur, baby food or many other things found in the grocery store.

I then explain that the only required element (my opinion) is some degree of dominance and at least a corresponding degree of submission for the scene to have all its most basic elements.

I have also heard the SM/leather encounter described in terms of music. The Top is the performer and the bottom as the instrument from which the performer tries to extract the most beautiful and satisfying "music." Each instrument has its particular limitations and wonders, and the performer's challenge and delight is to discover the capacities of the instrument he has chosen to play at the moment.

Others have described the experience in terms of sports like skydiving or bullfighting or scuba. Others think in terms of an outdoor adventure like a raft trip on a raging river. There are many ways to explain what the SM/leather experience is in terms of other experiences. With some thought and a careful assessment of your listener's capacities, you can break through the walls of ignorance that imprison us all, kinky and non-kinky alike.

A Leather Family?

"There is a reason my family does not know me and does not particularly want to know me any better than they do, and that reason is that I am very different from them. I am a leatherman, and they know it. Fortunately, I have another family, a much larger family of people who know, love, trust and respect me—my leather family. It is my most sincere wish that each of you will create for yourselves just such a supplemental family, because in these times when we are under attack from so many directions, we all need the support that can only come from such a family..."

—Guy Baldwin
International Mr. Leather contest, '89

Just what is a "leather family?" This is the group of people who care about us enough to share the important feelings and experiences that come with living life. For me, this always includes the leather/SM/fetish parts of myself.

With these people, we can be ourselves and not feel the need to hide the important parts of ourselves. They discover and like the fact that we are good people and that we have good intentions. They learn that we are not interested in destroying ourselves or others.

Since I know the most about my own leather family, it will be easiest to give readers a sense of what the experience is like if I describe my own impressions of these people and my relationships with them.

These are the people to whom I do not feel the need to lie even when my telling the truth places me in a poor light. I know that they care for me in spite of my flaws and shortcomings which I have revealed to them as time has passed. They love and appreciate my strengths and talents, and tolerate my weaknesses and smallness. They trust that I will grow into a better person because I want to.

Our values about what is important in life are similar enough to create respect and tolerance for those differences that inevitably emerge in all relationships. We cherish each other in different degrees at different times.

Members of my family know that I can be relied upon, and they understand that I may rely upon them at times. They come through for me as their resources permit; I come through for them as my resources permit. Without integrity, no such bond is possible.

Not all members of my family are equally resourceful—they are very different from each other. I do not try to borrow money from those who are poor—but they teach me about living simply. I don't make emotional demands on those dealing with disease—but they do teach me more about courage. I don't discuss politics with one of them; another is useless in affairs of the heart. But taken all together, they are a marvelous bunch of folks, and I accept the gifts of each, and respond with whatever feels right.

Over the years, many have died of various causes and, with each death, a hole was left in me and my family net. But, in time, I have met new people and they have become part of my ever-changing family. On rare occasion, I have lost a member of my leather family to the arms of drug addiction, usually after a great struggle. Whenever there is a profound change in values, family membership usually changes. This is true in all families; it is why I have become distant from my genetic family. Their values do not allow enough tolerance for my lifestyle.

Not all members of my leather family are acquainted with each other. Some have never met each other or, in a few cases, ever even heard of each other. Others spend time together often. I have frequent contact with some, occasional contact with others, and rare contact with a few others. But all would go to the wall for me to the extent of their resources in a pinch—this I know. All the members of my leather family are friends, but not all friends are "family." The twin forces of love and bonding are what makes the difference.

How are leather families "created?" The process begins with being honest with others about feelings. Many leathermen are poor at this because so many of us came from biological families where real feelings did not get talked about except perhaps under unusual circumstances.

As a result, many of us never learned how to share ourselves because we never saw Mom and Dad being open about themselves, except maybe when somebody had too much to drink, or there was a wedding or a funeral. Often, the rest of the time, everything was superficial. So we learned how to be superficial, too.

Being part of a leather family means learning how to be more than superficial. We learn how by not avoiding reality. This is hard to do sometimes. Participating in family life is not always easy, but it is deeply rewarding, and probably necessary in order for us to really flourish as people during tough times. It is also the best fun I have ever had.

How do we find people to be in our leather family? Well, you have to talk to people. This means choosing whom to talk with. Every leatherman you meet is a candidate for membership in your family until you disqualify him for whatever reason. Disqualification may happen immediately, or it may take some time. Most of us evaluate others all the time without thinking about it much—it seems to be a natural activity.

It will help to be clear about your ideas for what sort of people you want in your family. Whatever standards you apply to others will have to be applied to yourself also. For example, if you expect your family members to be reliable, then you won't be able to get away with being a flake yourself. Since you must tolerate flaws in yourself, you must also tolerate flaws in others. You will have to decide about which flaws are tolerable and which are not. You do this now but probably without thinking about it. To end up with a healthy leather family, you will do some thinking.

When you talk with someone initially, try to decide whether you want to become emotionally closer to the person or not. Keep your decision in mind as you continue your conversation. Watch for signs that he is interested in you, too. The interest need not be physical. Most of my family members don't turn me on sexually at all, and that's okay because that is not their purpose.

How do you find stuff to talk about? Everyone's life has pain in it. Everyone knows about fear. We all know about losses because we experience them from cradle to grave. But there are also feelings of joy and excitement, love and affection, jealousy and anger, all of which serve to create a balanced emotional life. These are the common personal experiences that bond people together in family networks based on mutual respect, love, interest, and integrity.

We can find out who the candidates for family are when we talk about these feelings with those we somehow suspect will understand and respond with support and acceptance. Then, we get to find out who is actually ready, willing and able to know us.

Of course, it works both ways: Is this person someone I am ready, willing and able to get to know? Being in a leather family is not just about receiving support, love and the rest; it also means a genuine need to participate in other people's lives just as they are participating in your own.

Because this is true, it is very helpful to sit down with yourself and notice your own ability to be in someone's family, too. If you are so self-preoccupied that there is no time or energy available except to manage your own work and living needs, then you may not have enough left over to contribute to being in a family. Unless there is something in the relationship for everybody, it won't work for long.

SM And Child Abuse:
For Some, A Difficult Connection
With The Past

CAUTION: The following article may stir up some serious emotional issues for some readers, especially those with child abuse in their backgrounds. If this is a touchy subject for you, you are advised to skip to the last paragraph for some suggested reading material which can ease you more gently into this subject.

For anyone paying attention to current issues in the news, child abuse has become a hot topic in the last several years. It is now estimated that as many as one woman in three and one man in five was physically and/or emotionally abused or sexually molested as a child. It is important for me to mention that the incidence of child abuse in the histories of practitioners of the SM/leather/fetish sexualities is astounding. While presenting seminars to leather folks, I have often asked how many in the room were subjected to child abuse as children, and I am still shocked when usually more than half the hands in the room go up.

Many survivors of child abuse (some simply don't survive) end up with a host of difficulties in their adult life that can be more or less directly traced to their abuse history.

These difficulties include, but are not limited to troubles forming intimate relationships, trouble with sexuality, trouble making new friends, trouble with people in the next older generation, and numerous other psychological problems.

In the therapy room, I frequently discover that SM bottoms are in the scene because they unconsciously try to recreate their

127

abusive experiences in the hopes that they can somehow un-do the traumas of their past and find love. During the SM scene itself, the bottom is returned to the emotional site of the original trauma back in time, but that is usually as far as it goes. Sometimes, things go a bit further when, after the bottom "breaks" in a scene, the Top moves closer emotionally to support the bottom. Then the desired "love" happens for the bottom. The irrational belief operating in bottom's head is, "If I can just get through this, the love will be waiting for me on the other side."

This sometimes resonates with messages the bottom may have received during abusive experiences as a child from a parent such as, "I'm only doing this for your own good," or "I'm doing this because I love you and I want you to turn out right." Tops with physical abuse in their childhood history can come at the SM scene from having made an identification with the abuser, so his (unconscious) belief can sound like this: "I'll show you my love the way that Dad (or Mom or whoever) showed me love (That is, I'll cause you pain)." Who can be surprised that love and abuse become emotionally linked together when children who received such treatment grow into adulthood?

Bottoms suddenly realize that something is wrong here when they first hear themselves say something like, "I get really uncomfortable when I meet a guy who is just too nice to me." The (conscious and aware) healthy part of them knows that that's just who they should be with, but the unhealthy (unconscious and unaware) part can't recognize such a person as a loving man without the abusive elements that remind them of childhood.

When the childhood abuse was sexual rather than physical or emotional, the child may grow up believing that sexual intimacy is love. In adulthood, these victims often run their sex lives ragged in the (unconscious) belief that sex equals love. They search for love in sex. But sex doesn't equal love, and so each sexual escapade leaves the adult feeling unfulfilled and depressed. They conclude (irrationally) that love didn't happen

128

because it wasn't the right guy, or that they didn't do the sex "right." And so they are driven to go out and try again with someone else. They become sexual compulsives.

I know that my comments here will anger some who feel that I am playing into the hands of the psychiatric view that all SM is a maladaptive response to child abuse. But I have learned that in *some* cases, that view is correct. I also know that some will be annoyed at my opposition to the SM elements of anger and humiliation in the playroom, but I have reason to suspect that anger and humiliation in the playroom often signal the unconscious attempt to recreate the emotional environment of childhood abuse. While it is true that people have a right to play the way they wish, I cannot support what I feel amounts to the ongoing abuse of the inner child. At the same time, I recognize that people have a right to hang on to behaviors that don't work and don't make them feel better.

Clearly, not all adult survivors of child abuse end up in the SM scene; if that were the case, the SM scene would be much larger than it appears to be. Likewise, not everyone in the SM scene is there to unconsciously work out his child abuse issues, but I am convinced that some percentage of us are there for just this purpose. But the SM scene, even with all it's glories, does not have the power or ability to accomplish the psychological restructuring that is necessary to really heal the wounds suffered during childhood. At best, it can only offer a setting for the recreation of the abusive environment, and then apply a BandAid. At worst, it doesn't even offer the BandAid.

The SM scene does offer the opportunity to transform consciousness and stimulate ecstatic erotic catharsis. And even though SM can sometimes feel psychologically refreshing, that is not the same thing as the psychological restructuring of psychotherapy. SM should never be expected to heal the wounded inner child who doesn't belong in the playroom in the first place. SM is for consenting adults only, and when we bring our wounded inner children into an SM scene, we are only continuing the abuses of the past, reinforcing depression, and prolonging a frustrated search for love.

Here are some books that can help shed more light on recovering from child abuse: *Victims No More* by Mike Lew; Harper & Row, 1988, 1990. This book is a good place to start. It focuses on abused males specifically. Read slowly, and take this one in very small bites. *The Courage To Heal Workbook* by Laura Davis; Harper & Row, 1990. This is a very practical, step-by-step approach to healing. *Homecoming: Reclaiming and Championing Your Inner Child* by John Bradshaw; Bantam Books, 1990. A good book to finish up with.

Beauties & Beasts Revisited

Recently, an article titled "The Beauties & The Beasts" was brought to my attention by someone who thought I might find it interesting, and because my name appears in it. For those readers who may have missed this thoughtful and provocative article, I shall offer my imperfect summary before I comment on it.

The author asserted that the leather community suffers from a terminal condition he describes as a split between the younger, handsome, in good physical shape, shallow, depressed leather beauties who have insecurities about their inner selves, and the older, wiser, brighter, educated, but dumpy men whose assets are intangible. The guys in both groups, he contends, are frustrated and somehow incomplete, and each needs the assets of the other to achieve inner harmony.

The proposed solution to this state of affairs is to establish networks in the community which encourage the development of partnerships composed of one beauty and one beast, so that each can supply guidance and inspiration for the something the other one needs. He seems to feel that such partnerships will produce more balance in the lives of both beauties and beasts. It's a fine idea.

The article is clear that these relationships need not be sexual, and reminds us of our history of "brotherhood" during the bike club era, when beauties were thrown together with beasts under common banners.

Interestingly enough, the article points to me as a "rare" example of a leatherman with both the "magnificent" physical gifts he associates with the young muscle beauties and the considerable non-physical talents he associates with the beasts.

"I wonder if he had a younger man to help him in this [body building]," the author asks in his article. He must know

131

that I am, or was (?), a "beast."

The answer is, 5% yes, and 95% no. It should come as no surprise to anyone who knows me that I learned the body stuff mostly from books where it is available to anyone in twenty languages ("beasts" take note). And with this, I shall begin to outline my variance with the author's ideas about our community's ailments.

But perhaps "variance" is not quite the right word. I do agree that it would be nice if beauties and beasts gave more to each other, but I feel that way about humanity in general. I suspect that the paradoxes of the respective beauty/beast psychologies will probably continue to prevent much of the needed change from happening. The article even discusses some of the internal processes that paralyze the beauties/beasts, stopping their movement toward integration of their respective missing parts.

But I have some problems with the assumptions the article seems to be based upon. First off, the mere suggestion that the beautiful, young, well-built guys that one sees in the bars and in the magazines are vapid air heads is an insult. It is simply not true. While the so called beasts have had their noses in books, the world has changed. More attractive, bright, young leather guys, some with professional accomplishments, have been coming out, and many of them have no fear about posing nude for a photo spread, or discussing Dante or Heisenberg in a leather bar.

In short, to imagine that the lives of the beautiful, muscle built young men are hollow is often what the beasts want to believe, if only to more easily justify their sedentary "life of the mind," and one more piece of fudge.

The flip side of these facts is that it is also not true that men with grey hair and experience of life are all in terrible physical shape. Each year's International Mr. Leather competition and many other major leather events I attend clearly demonstrate that many leather men have rejected the outdated notion that over 40 means over the hill.

The impressive contestants in another international leather

contest—Mr. Drummer 1990—included an architect, a social worker, two teachers and a lawyer, all with grey hair and bodies very few would throw out of bed or playroom. During the interviews, they revealed great depth of character to match their physical prowess.

My message here is that role models exist for the notion of an integrated personality and physicality at any age. While the idea of shallow and lost beauties teamed up with wise and unfulfilled beasts may sound attractive to those who fit the descriptions, I fear the consequences for both members of any such team. My guess, speaking as a psychotherapist now, is that such unions would run the risk of becoming co-dependant and thereby actually stunt the growth of both.

Two "half" people do not make a whole person; they make two halves of two persons. I am much more attracted to the idea of people becoming whole; self-contained and self-sufficient; balanced between mind and body through their own efforts. Therapists of all persuasions understand the danger that arises when anyone, "beauty" or "beast," thinks that someone else can fix whatever is wrong, or supply what is missing in their lives.

In my own case, if I had waited for some young man to teach me about body things it would have been one hell of a long wait. And now, I would not be able to take full credit for my achievement. No one lifts the weight for us, *ever*. Indeed, I think it is wise to distrust anyone who promises to "lift the weight" for you. That person does not want your freedom; he wants your dependence, and craves your endless gratitude and devotion.

I suspect that the article under discussion is really supporting the idea of a kind of mutual mentoring, but I fear that people will be attracted to the suggestion for beauty/beast teams because they look like a way *around* having to "lift the weight" for oneself. This is the reason that the "eat anything you like" diets sell so well. Lots of people just simply don't want to do the hard work that goes with becoming a healthy and well rounded human being.

No one, including myself, is suggesting that such work is easy or even fast. I have spent over five years struggling with my body, trying to make some muscles, and a good deal longer struggling with my mind trying to train it to think and feel. Too bad. It takes what it takes.

If you want to get what is in a book, you have to go through all the pages line by line. This may even mean learning how to read, and I know that most beasts are not qualified reading teachers.

Transforming beast bodies is an equally complex process often requiring a sophisticated knowledge of metabolism that I know few beauties possess since they usually have no need for such data. If you want a body that is attractive to yourself, that means digging for the needed information and, one day at a time, doing the god damned work, while figuring out how to make it fun.

Doing so is much less mysterious that you might think. There are more and more men over 40 in fitness programs precisely because the fitness people realized that this market was going untapped. Fitness videos are now widely available so that one can get started in the privacy of one's own home. Gym owners have seen their marketing problem too, and so they are now more welcoming to those of us who are middle aged than was once the case.

Qualified (usually younger) guys are available (yes, for a fee) to share their knowledge with those who want to take the body project seriously, whether that means muscles, or slimming down and toning up. Let's not turn up our noses at paying these guys a fee—we all sell whatever we know best to earn a living. Let him who is not, by this definition, a prostitute cast the first stone.

In fact, there is more support today for us "beasts" getting fit than ever before. Please be clear that by "fit" I mean not just physically fit, but also the added bonus of physical self confidence and respect that goes with fitness. This support includes a host of well written books on the subject. The time for living in fear and denial about our deficiencies has passed.

134

Beasts, start getting fit now. It will never be easier than it is today.

As for the beauty or beast whose life feels empty, most of his work will, understandably, be on his inside self. Most of the emotionally shallow folks I have met suffer from the inability to look steadily inward. It hurts too much. Perhaps the single most fearsome obstacle to becoming a whole person that any of us faces is drug abuse, always including alcohol, of course.

This is probably because drugs offer temporary relief for the unwelcome feelings of pain that always accompany self exploration. Drugs appear to offer a way around the pain. When used, real self exploration always seems to halt.

When drugs are not an option for relief, beauties will often try to escape the pain of the self explorations that lead to inner maturity by running away into physical activity. Likewise the beast in similar flight often escapes into intellectual pursuits, a food addiction, or perhaps his work. In whichever case, real self exploration also grinds to a halt.

Put simply, the beauties have to do one kind of work to become well balanced, and the beasts have to do another kind of work. While it is easy for anyone to lay back and grouse about the lack of community support for becoming well rounded, time is steadily passing. Whatever else we might think about them, the Act Up people are right about something when they say, "Action = Life." And so it does.

None of us can afford to wait one more day until the right teacher presents himself for us to tap as a resource. It is dangerous for anyone to wait for guides to lead us into the happier world we wish for ourselves, though we do need to be sensitive to real mentoring relationships when they present themselves. Whether we like it or not, no one is likely to knock at our door and offer to take us by the hand to the local gym or library.

We must each accept the personal responsibility for our own growth into the fullness of a healthy and well balanced adulthood. Anything less is just prolonged adolescence, and this essential choice is perhaps the real issue.

Leather In The '90s:
Another View

I just read an article in which the writer discussed in the previous essay articulates very clearly some of the malaise that has developed in the leather scene. He went further, to assert that "leather died" in the 1980s. I do not agree. Having traveled some 40,000 miles to visit with leathermen in 25 cities during the past two years (1989-90), I can reassure you that, while some things are troublesome, the fire that drives us will never be extinguished because it is in our souls. Talk of ashes and phoenix rising may sound romantic, but it is premature at best and defeatist at worst to suggest that leather is dead.

As is usual with this particular writer, he seems to be searching for solutions to today's problems in the traditions of the Old Guard past. Resurrecting bygone attitudes in the search for solutions to present troubles can be risky because our world has changed so much.

Reading the suggestions that leathermen should buy and ride motorcycles, that rubbermen should take up scuba diving, and so on, took me right back to 1965. I recall quite well how the riding guys looked down on non-riders, and those without motorcycles felt self-conscious about getting out of their cars wearing full leather.

There was a clear premium placed on "authenticity." So called "real" leathermen were supposed to be the ones who rode Harleys (not Hondas) and didn't talk much about much. Working class guys, especially those who worked with their hands outdoors were somehow the "real" thing and therefore more desirable—to have sex with, that is; or to have fantasies about. These were the "real" men who did "real" work and had "real" sex. Problem was, it often turned out that they weren't "real" interesting people, and often had no erotic imagination and got boring fast once the sex was over. I also recall that they hated minorities and anyone who was sensitive and didn't look like themselves.

I guess this writer wants the rubber lover in Iowa to move to San Diego and take scuba lessons in spite of his heart condition or else keep his interest in rubber private. Likewise, I guess I was not a real leatherman before I bought my Harley in 1982, and I should now turn in my credentials since I sold the bike in April, 1990, to help finance my fund raising travels. Now I drive to local events in my VW.

I was particularly amused to read the objections to stacked riding heels on the cowboy boots of horseless men. Having grown up in western Colorado on a ranch, I know the writer is right about the purpose of the stacked heels. They are safer and easier to ride with, and were not made for walking. I don't ride horses anymore, but, and here is my point: riding heels make my dick hard! And that, frankly, is what the sexual part of my leatherhood is really all about.

To quote the author, "Reality is, and must be, based on truth." I agree, and the truth is that men who love to wear uniforms, need not become cops to justify their interests. The bottom line with the sexual part of the leather scene must be determined by what makes our brains and dicks hard. It is dangerous to one's sexual identity to be "other" directed. We do not need Leather Fashion Police to tell us how to dress; we can get that guidance from between our legs just fine. Fashion rules, no matter who makes them, are part of the "extra baggage we can do without in the '90s" and beyond.

There are some great traditions associated with the Old Guard: loyalty and brotherhood just to name two. But all that old condescension towards outsiders, and all that fascination with being "authentic," only slowed guys down in the search for their true erotic selves.

I sincerely want to encourage bankers who are leather lovers to wear their leather shamelessly and with pride wherever and whenever they want, whether they like motorcycles or not. I advise the same freedom for all other fetishists and erotically different folks.

The answers to what ails our scene will be found in the future, not in the past. Yes, there are good things back there, but there was a lot of chaff mixed in with that wheat, and it is our job to fearlessly examine our traditions to preserve what worked, and replace what did not with new ideas. My experience has shown me that there are many different ways to jack off, make love, be a leatherman, arrange flowers, and do any other damn thing you care to name. Lifestyle intolerance is part of the problem, not part of the solution.

I was more than a little surprised by the author's question, "Why is no one working to change things and create some fresh options (in the leather scene)?" Where has he been? Does he read all the classified ads in leather/SM magazines? There are now hundreds of clubs and organizations in this country and overseas. Just here in the U.S., the clubs range from the traditional bike clubs to groups (clans?) catering to those into mud (Club Mud), cigars (Hot Ash), piercing (PFI), tatoos (Illustrated Men), boots, whips, ad infinitum. These groups were put together for exactly the reasons the writer now urges their creation: to facilitate contact between fetishists with similar interests in non-bar settings that provide mutual support. Even a cursory glance at any of the comprehensive calendars of leather events will reveal quickly that there is a wealth of contact opportunity available outside leather bars for those who are interested.

To suggest that no one is working on options is an insult to the endless hard work that goes on all over this country to develop new institutions in support of those people, young and old, who are getting more honest with themselves about all their needs and not just the sexual ones either. If, as the article suggests, "...Leather men are left isolated in their homes or apartments with no place to meet," it is often because they are unwilling to participate in the growing network that is available to them, and it must be their choice to participate or not. The article is right when it makes the point that modern leathermen will get out of the scene just what they are willing to put into it.

Perhaps I talk to more people than the writer does (he admits to being stuck on the sidelines) but, unlike him, I hear many success stories about people meeting on phone lines, over computers or through ads in various publications. These, too, are new and fresh institutions that were not available in the past, and now offer leather folks new opportunities for contact and support.

Recently, I was (again) privileged to serve as a judge at the Mr. Mid-Atlantic Leather contest. If the author of the article under discussion had been there, he would have witnessed in one weekend many manifestations of all the things he feels are missing from the leather scene today: participation by 79 quite varied clubs and organizations from many states and five foreign countries; a beautiful and highly ritualized passing of the flame from one set of leadership to another; 19 highly motivated contestants (aged 24-53) with ideals of brotherhood, community service, records of service achievement both in and out of the leather scene; a real commitment to improving the quality of life in the leather scene; a speech about the value of ritual in our daily lives delivered by Mark Ryan, aged 24, then serving as International Mr. Leather 1990. and much more.

While it is certainly true that once upon a time all winners of leather contests were merely two-dimensional erotic icons, things have changed in most places. Most titleholders last year (1990) assisted greatly in raising hundreds of thousands of dollars (yes!) for a wide variety of AIDS related purposes, local community newspapers, efforts to unseat Jesse Helms, and many other worthy causes. We have stood on countless stages and urged leather folks everywhere to develop family-type groups for their own support and development. Today, most contest judges are unwilling to select contestants who can't or won't continue along these paths. To my eye, this looks like "males who have shouldered the responsibilities of adulthood." Occasionally, a loser does get past the judges at a contest, but the trend toward choosing meaningful role models is clear for anyone to see, anyone who is willing to make an effort to follow these things.

The article is right to suggest that "we will have to start with the basics." From where I stand, that means paying attention to what is between our legs, our ears and our elbows. For myself, I much prefer the scene as it is in 1991 to what it was in 1965. Now, there is lots of information available about any erotic activity you care to name, and easy ways to get it. That was not true in 1965 when the Old Guard was into secrets. Nowadays, no one is forced to go to bars to meet their counterparts if that is not their scene. These days, someone age 27 is likely to be just as knowledgeable about any particular part of the leathersex scene as someone 57, if not more so. There has never been more ritual process available than today. Many leather events across the nation feel more like family reunions than did the drunken camp-outs that describe most "bike runs" of the '60s and '70s.

Yes, there are problems, but none so great as the cynicism and backward looking melancholy I hear and read about from those who are, and choose to remain, out of step with what is really happening in the scene today. Today's leather scene offers more real nourishment to seekers than has ever been available before. There will always be people in bars and other settings who turn us off for whatever reason. So what! If we can keep ourselves moving steadily toward what works for us personally, and adds to our lives as a whole, then life will work better for us. The alternative is to allow ourselves to be constantly distracted and annoyed by those who don't happen to turn us on, or are just into adolescent posing.

It is the job of those responsible for leadership in the community to develop and maintain nourishing institutions in the leather scene so that when the adolescent poseurs tire of themselves, they will have something of substance to be guided by if they so choose. This job will require more than cynical carping. It calls for commitment and consistent participation in the evolution of the lifestyle. It calls for love and patience.

141

Political Scat
Or, Is There Really Anything
But The Smell?

Some months ago, the publisher asked me to write an article about leather community politics. Since he is a kindly fellow and well-intentioned, I agreed and promised to submit an outline of my ideas in a few days. But many weeks passed, and my guilt about not following through with my promise grew until I was forced to confront the fact that I was reluctant to do the project. The reason: I realize that what I have to say here won't be very popular with most of the so called "movers and shakers." But this—Fall, 1992—has been the season for politics in general, so I figure that now is as good a time as any for sticking our noses in some reality—at least reality as I have come to see it.

To begin with, I have problems with the whole notion of a "leather community." I'm not at all sure that one exists in any meaningful or useful sense of the word. I intend for this article to cause us to reconsider the idea altogether.

In the first place, "leather" is a euphemism. As we use it, it can mean motorcycle riders, SM practitioners, leather fetishists, uniform fetishists, rubber fetishists—in fact, fetishists of many sorts—lovers of "rough sex," or simply butch looking types. Even within these groups, things are different depending on whether one is a gay man, a lesbian, heterosexual, bi-sexual, or a transgenderal person. Put each of these various types together in the same room, and I guarantee that very few of them will be comfortable with everyone else there.

That doesn't exactly sound like "community" to me. But then, not all Republicans like each other either, yet they still feel connected enough to work together. (I guess it must be easier when the things that connect you happen above your neck rather than below your waist.)

Secondly, the relevant definition of "community" for this discussion is: a social group sharing common characteristics or interests and which is perceived or perceives itself as distinct in some respect from the larger society within which it exists.

One of the many reasons that I wanted the job of International Mr. Leather in 1989 was to have the opportunity to get a look at the national "leather community" up close. I wanted to see just what characteristics or interests we shared. (Naive me,) I was startled to discover that on a geographic basis alone, there were actually more like 15 leather communities all across the continent, and that each one reflected the regional attitudes and norms of their area. Today, I am less provincial in my views.

In conservative states, leather folks tended to have conservative attitudes, and liberal attitudes prevailed in liberal regions. The leather men in Quebec will never forgive me for using the word "Canada" in a speech. Some Texans were shocked that I was personally pro-choice. New Yorkers were uncomfortable with my direct eye-contact and direct questions. Bostonians were put off by my easy-going California style. Spiritual issues seem generally more important to those of us in the West, while such things are often dismissed as being "too California" in the East. In Washington, DC, statehood was a big issue because those people have such a strange relationship with Congress. In short, leather was not the tie that binds.

I was even startled to learn that different regions have different attitudes about doing leather sex itself. In some places, bottoms are seen as second class citizens, in others, they are prized. Even with all the traveling, national-level teachers giving seminars and workshops, there are still widely divergent attitudes about style.

In short, even though leather folks look pretty much the same from place to place, beneath the surface, big differences still exist in consciousness, technical skill, psychological sophistication, their attitudes toward themselves, their erotic

144

interests, and so forth. Finally, I came to the conclusion that the only thing that almost all of us share is an interest in erotic experiences involving dominance and submission and/or certain fetishes. In theory, that should be enough to make a community. In practice, it doesn't seem to.

Now, I'll come to the politics part. First, the leaders.

For better or for worse, there is a *very small* group of leather folks who have a passionate commitment to see things change in this country, at least with respect to the treatment of erotic minorities. People who are passionate enough to speak out consistently, and have social change as their goal are very rare.

These people can be roughly divided into four groups: (some) leather titleholders; (some) club affiliated activists; (some) non-affiliated independents; and (some) artists. Those in the first group are chosen by a small handful of judges who can be found on the contest circuit. Those in the second group are generally elected by club membership, and those in the last two groups are self-appointed.

Additionally, titleholders and elected spokespersons have built-in term limits—usually, they serve for only one year. The down side of this fact is that those with good things to say don't get to hang around long enough to promote their ideas to maturity. The upside is that we don't have to put up with airhead do-nothing people for very long.

But in any case, erotic politics have a very narrow idea base in that, when all the right things have been said, the only thing left to do with them is repeat them with more creative packaging. After a while, this gets old. People stop listening, and apathy grows. "Yes, yes, we've heard it all before." Until we decide to run a candidate for local, state or national office, I'm not sure there is very much more for our political leaders to say. Any new people that come out into the leather scene can now find it all in print, if they are really interested, that is.

If the future for leather folks can be predicted from the gay and lesbian experience, then it stands to reason that the most important and first steps will be the development of new

145

consciousness among ourselves. Stonewall did that for the gay mainstream in the late '60s.

The next really important thing that happened was that the American Psychiatric Association took homosexuality out of their list of mental disorders in 1973. We aren't even close to having that happen for us, *yet*. These two events were necessary before the legal establishment could begin to slowly reconsider the social position of homosexuals. Then more gays and lesbians started to come out, and some began to run for public office, and get elected. Slowly, the stigma of homosexuality has begun to erode. But the fact is that the vast majority of homosexuals have not been much a part of this process *at all*. And so it is with leather folks. Besides, there are far fewer of us, so it is reasonable to expect that things will go slower for us.

As a group, leather folks are about where mainstream gay and lesbian people were in 1970. We are still regarded as mentally disordered by the psychological world. Legally, we have practically no protections whatever. This is what most leather leaders want to see change.

Incidentally, the so-called leather leadership role is not to be had without a price. I know of no leather community leaders who haven't spent huge sums out of their own pockets to get out and make their opinions known. Collectively, the holders of the International Mr. Leather title from 1985 to 1991 spent somewhere in the neighborhood of $40,000.00 of their own money to "do the job." Almost all International Ms. Leather titleholders have faced bankruptcy to get their messages out. The democratically elected leaders of the leather community do not enjoy financial support from their own organizations for travel and other associated costs. Essentially, leadership is done for love and, sometimes, a bit of short-lived glory. Burnout is common.

In general, there is little, if any, real accountability for the actions of these leaders. They have no real authority, have widely divergent agendas, and with the exception of one titleholder, and the officers of some major organizations, report

146

to no one about their activities.

There is no single forum where these leaders meet to establish policy or thrash out issues, and an attempt to establish such a forum sputtered into forgotten silence in 1990. Occasional efforts by the National Leather Association to have leadership forums during their annual Living in Leather conferences have been weakened by sparse attendance.

The closest thing we have to any such forum exists in the publications which print the views of various leaders. The publications themselves are not widely read, are expensive to read on a regular basis, and contain little information of interest to everyone with the single exception of the classified ads. (That was a hint.)

To make matters worse, the leaders occasionally find themselves engaged in turf wars or ideological disputes, which sometimes find their way into the public eye. When this happens, it creates the impression that there is ideological disarray and that leaders are missing the big picture. It is easy not to pay attention to squabblers.

Now, on to the followers, the rank and file people in this so-called community: In spite of the fact that wearing leather or otherwise engaging in SM/fetish behavior is, itself, a kind of political statement, *as a group*, leather people are not particularly political on that basis alone. Most leather folks just plain don't give a damn about leather politics, the social position of perverts, our relationship to the larger mainstream gay/lesbian community, and the lot. Hell, it is even tough to get most leather folks excited about the censorship of so called pornography—something that reaches underneath our very own beds!

So, we are left with what appears to me to be an altogether silly situation: mostly unaccountable "leaders" trying to motivate a politically disinterested and very diverse group of people who would really just rather get laid. In fact, getting laid consumes much more of our time, energy and financial resources than anything else connected with our erotic life.

Here is some more evidence for you to chew on. The

largest annual gathering of leather folks that I know of is the International Mr. Leather weekend in Chicago. Several thousand leather folks (95% gay men) travel to Chicago that weekend, but most don't bother to go to the contest itself. They gather in Chicago primarily to be with their own kind mostly in the bars, which are always packed.

As for the contest itself, the highlight of the evening (at least as measured by crowd response) isn't the speeches, which are essentially political and motivational in nature. It is the "jockstrap" portion in which the contestants show skin, and get seductive with the audience. And who can really be surprised? This is, after all, at base, an erotic thing that we are into.

Like it or not, getting horny can drive the most noble political thought right out of almost any brain. Brain chemistry is like that. It's been that way for a very long time simply because Mother Nature is more interested in our sex drive than in damn near anything else. Most of us would rather cruise than march on Washington, DC. On the other hand, at a really big rally, the cruising can be great, and it's good politics, too.

I'm tired of this article, and I'm going out to see if the evening holds any excitement.

Part Three

ON ENHANCING THE SM EXPERIENCE

Editor's Note On
On Enhancing The SM Experience

Nothing I might add to this section by way of introducing it could be more important than this: Do not mistake these essays for basic SM instructions. How-to books are being published, but this is not one of them. The words with which Baldwin chose to title the section mean exactly what they say, placing the emphasis on enhancement not instruction.

The first essay in this part of the book, "You Go Together, Or You Don't Go At All," is the only piece in the book that comprises more than one previously published article. Baldwin had explored the subject of communication between SM partners in three closely related articles. They overlapped. They refused to be fitted in any order. They would not behave as separate essays, no matter how I cajoled or abused them. Then, like magic, the three articles snapped together into one essay. If I have weakened Baldwin's arguments, I can only apologize, adding in my own defense that this essay works *for me*.

The remainder of the section deals with Tops and bottoms, drugs, and SM mind sets. The subjects are more distinct from one another—at a certain level—than is the case in other sections of the book. Nonetheless, I believe, the reader who keeps in mind the purpose and title of the section will be able to knit these essays together very usefully.

In dealing with important aspects of what can go wrong in a scene, and how to avoid having things go wrong, Baldwin often repeats themes and ideas. This reiteration has not been completely edited out because the information is worthy of repetition *and* because the essays need to remain separately readable, each bearing the burden of its own intent just as it did when first published in a magazine.

You Go Together, Or You Don't Go At All!

One of the many wonderful and satisfying things about being in an SM relationship is that there is so much less time spent looking for someone to play with—he is often in the next room. But if the process of sexual communications has broken down, we are usually left with the feeling of, "So near, and yet so far away."

The partnerships that I have seen working well erotically have developed a process of communication about sex that is mutually supportive, and that leads them steadily toward the horizons of their fantasy life. Satisfaction in the various SM sexualities comes with practice, and to make scenes in partnerships really wonderful requires a cooperative effort. Usually, they get better only when our learning becomes cumulative—builds on itself. For this to happen, partnerships need the skills that can help refine their sex together, so it gets them where they want to go. There are a number of these communication skills that you can learn and use to move your partnership in the erotic directions that are mutually satisfying.

I want to present some suggestions for the development of these skills. These are ideas that have come to me while working in the therapy room with guys who just haven't been able to get the erotic parts of their relationship working as smoothly as they might have liked. Not all the suggestions will apply to your situation, so take what seems to fit and ignore the rest for now. You may be able to use more some other time.

Basically the skills divide themselves nicely into three categories: what you can, even *must* discuss before the first scene; what you may need to discuss between scenes, meaning before the next one; and what is communicated during an SM scene.

Already, I know that I run the risk of pissing off a whole bunch of people who will yell that I have no right to tell them how to communicate when they play. They are right—I don't! I have said elsewhere that there are many right ways to do SM, and I stand by that. It is also true that there are many wrong ways to do SM, and one of them involves unwillingness or inability to "take care of business" before the scene happens.

Before the First Scene

For the first scene between strangers, there are, in my opinion, some essential types of information that must be exchanged if the scene is to have a reasonable chance of being a special experience for both players. People looking for relationships with SM partners will often want to repeat scenes when they have gone well.

At the top of this list of essential communications is agreement about safer sex practices if any sort of penetration or other juicy activities (wet) are even a remote possibility or wish for either partner.

I believe it is unwise to deal with this issue "as the scene progresses," because once things get moving, passions (drugs and alcohol too) can and do cloud judgement for both Tops and bottoms. Also, experienced Tops know how unsettling it is to be in the middle of something and have to deal with an interruption from a bottom who is scared about catching "it" from something he is about to do. So, I suggest that you have this conversation before you start to play, unless you are willing to risk your life on your ability to handle these issues when you are horny, and maybe also stoned.

This goes for everyone. Those who play in Podunk and think they are exempt from this issue are not thinking with their brains, but with their dicks which have one track minds. In Podunk or Metropolis, strangers who tell you they are "negative" may be lying, and it is dangerous to assess a man's credibility when you are horny and about to play.

Unfortunately, many of you avoid the subject of safer sex

154

because you have not yet learned how to bring it up. Thinking about safer sex conversations just before a scene makes most men nervous, so the tendency is to deal with the issues as you go along, if at all.

Some men only barely mention it and secretly hope that the subject changes soon. Bottoms worry that bringing the subject up is somehow "un-bottom-like," and that doing so might turn the Top off. That won't do anymore.

Since most SM players are already used to negotiating their sex play anyway, safer sex just becomes one more thing to be talked about before the decision to play is made. Remember this fact to help calm your nerves about these conversations.

Here are a few ideas about how to manage this matter. As you read them, remember that it is useless to memorize my words—they are mine, not yours. Yours will be better. It will help more if you remember the gist of the attitude, or the tone the words carry.

A bottom might say: "I know that I will be easier to play with after we have agreed about safer sex things," or maybe, "I will be too scared to play until you have made some promises about not swapping fluids," or "It will help me to be with you more comfortably when I have heard your thoughts about Aids safety," or "What are your rules about sex between us?" or "Can we do SM without having any actual sex?" or "I want to play, but there are only certain ways it will be OK for us to have actual sex together. I need to talk about them first."

Or, how about these approaches from the bottom: "I hope to serve you well without risking my health, Sir." "I can play harder and heavier if I don't have to worry all the time about watching to see if you are about to do something with me that is unhealthy. I guess we should talk more first." "I can't deal with a hood if I am scared that you might do anything unhealthy with me." "I know that you are a very experienced player, and I hope you won't be insulted by my asking, but can we have some conversation first about healthy ways to do this." Or, finally, "Aside from the standard safe sex rules, what else are you into these days, Mister?" (My thanks to A.K. for this last one.)

A Top might say: "We're going to play, but we're not going to do anything that might endanger either your health or mine," or, "I expect you to take some risks, but not to risk your life or mine," or "I do like to fuck, but only with a rubber, and I always pull out before I cum" or "Since you haven't mentioned it yet, I will. I don't swap fluids nohow, so if that's what you might be hoping for, forget it," or "You are not to get near my cock unless I say so, Got it?" Perhaps adding the assurance that, "you can be damn sure that if my cock touches you that it will be in the grip of rubber first."

Or, a Top might make safer sex conversation part of the onset of the scene itself by ordering it: "You will now slowly and carefully outline for me your notions of what is and is not sexually safe, and what you are scared about around exposure to the viruses we are all concerned about."

My point here is that there are lots of ways to initiate such a conversation. Anyone who is unwilling or unable to tolerate such talk cannot be presumed to be Safe, Sane and Consensual.

Realize that before you can be a full participant in such a conversation, you must get familiar with the current thinking about what is and is not safe to do. Unfortunately, there is some middle ground about the subject of safety, especially around oral sex, which only makes familiarity with the current information even more important.

Everyone must determine what activities they are and are not willing to enjoy, and how they intend to protect their health and the health of their partners. If you are relationship oriented, then part of your task will be to identify those men who share your views about safer sex. Staying alive and healthy is a fine basis on which to found a new relationship.

Before the Next Scene

Sometime before you play again, preferably days before, it is usually a good idea to have some conversation about the last scene, or the last few scenes that you have had. These conversations can work well as mealtime talks because you are already taking another kind of nourishment together. It's smart to choose a time that is emotionally un-charged for both of you—for everyone, if you are a trio, quartet, or larger family arrangement. Trying to talk about intimate feelings connected to sexuality when tempers are running hot is generally not helpful. It is sometimes too tempting to use what doesn't work sexually as a weapon or bargaining chip during an argument.

Your agenda for this sort of conversation is to try to say what worked for you and what did not, and, if you know, why not. Your other agenda is to support the next scene happening. So you might hear remarks like: "Did that scene last Friday gettcha where you live?" or "I had fun with you that night, and I know you had fun too. What did you like best about it?" or "Y'know, last week when we played, what happened was upsetting for me, and I guess it was for you too. How do we avoid that happening next time?" or "Is there some way you can think of that would have made our last scene work better for you?" or, "Thanks for a great time last Tuesday morning. It was the best! It was hot when you..."

Talking about sex is not easy for this entire society, and it is even tougher for kinky people to do because there are no models for this. Whatever you do, please remember to be kind to each other when you talk about sex together. We are all pretty sensitive about these things, you know.

When trying to talk about your scenes, it may be helpful to follow these guidelines:

1) Tell the truth. Now, there are many ways to tell the truth about something. Your words must be chosen very carefully when you are talking about sex with your SM partner, because the words you choose may hurt his feelings which (hopefully) is not your purpose. Hurt feelings do *not* support the next scene happening. Remember! Your purpose is to make SM better for yourself, not to piss each other off. Your conversation will be a failure unless you both get to exchange information that will be valuable for the next scene! Lies only complicate things, and will have to be corrected sooner or later. Lies make for secrets,

and secrets—especially about sex—can make for terrible trouble.

2) Stress cooperation. If you stop to think about it, a Top and bottom in a relationship form a kind of erotic team. As with all teams, there are problems to be solved. Everybody wants to win. The best sexual "win" is when everyone gets where they need to go. Solutions that don't work for both (all) partners don't work *period*.

Example: "When I whip you, I always wish you could take more. Maybe you could tell me if you think there is a way for me to do it that would increase your tolerance, because that is something I would like us to develop together if we can. I need your help with this." Without criticism, the remark reveals a disappointment for the Top. It also tells the bottom plainly what the Top needs, and that he wants the bottom's help to make it happen. If the bottom is listening carefully, he will hear that the Top *needs* him on the team. You go together, or you don't go.

3) Don't criticize! Make reports about yourself instead. This means that you don't tell him not to do something, instead you tell him about your response to his behavior. So you get, "When you close your eyes, it feels like you want to get away from me. Do you?" or, "I like it better when you keep your eyes open." The critical, and therefore inappropriate alternative is, "You always close your eyes at the wrong time."

Another example: "When you whip me real hard from the start, I don't have a chance to get my head into it," instead of "I hate the way you whip me." And another: "When you wear your sneakers, I don't get turned on to playing with you," instead of "You look like a fag when you wear those things, wear boots next time." Or, "Although I like being with you very much, it was easier to get hot together before you picked up these last 35 pounds. Playing is still great for me until it comes to dealing with all your extra flesh—it is not hot for me." This is factual information about real feelings, but is not critical.

4) Try to give a balanced report. Don't turn your feedback into a "shit" list. It is perhaps more important to say what you

loved than it is to say what you hated. Sexual feedback is really the process of supporting what you like in your partner, and trying to modify what you don't like. Remember, there are lots of ways to tell the truth: "I love it when you bring your face close to mine, and talk the way you do. I would like it better still if I smelled mouthwash (or a cigar, or whatever) on your breath." But not, "Your breath stinks and is a soft-on!"

Or, it might be necessary to say, "I like the Idea of you with a cigar, but not the smell of them. Can we look for a brand that we both will like?" It is not necessary to say, "I have always hated the way the damn things smell."

More examples: "If you want me to get hard when you tie me up, I should probably tell you the chances are better when you tie things tighter." Or, "It will be difficult for me to whip you harder unless I hear you beg me for more, because I worry about going too far with you. Besides, it turns me on when you beg for it."

5) In technical discussions, don't be afraid to be specific. Say, "It worked great up until you did such and such, then I started to have problems. Maybe if so and so happens first, it might work better next time." Or, "The big one is just too distracting for me unless you start with the smaller one, and go slower. I want the big one, but I think I need to work up to it."

Or, "When I have you tied up with the dingus, would you deal with it longer if the whatsit part wasn't so tight" or "I know you get scared when I put on the blindfold and can't play as hard. What if it had small pin holes in it to let light through to you, but were too small for me to see, cuz I luv how you look blindfolded."

6) Consider introducing activities that you are interested in exploring. There are gentle ways to do this: "Have you ever done X, and was it any fun?" Or, "I read a story about X once, and it scared me and turned me on at the same time." Or, "I did so and so once with a guy. It could have been interesting if he had done it differently."

There are also not-so-gentle ways to do this: "I am good at fisting, and love to do it. I want us to do that. I know what

159

precautions to take. Have you ever been fisted, and how?" Or, "I want us to learn about whips (or bondage or whatever), and I want us to start talking about it a lot first."

7) Try to keep these conversations short at first, till you feel comfortable with the process, and have settled into a style for talking that seems successful. Try to experiment with this. One couple I worked with took to writing notes to each other, and it worked!

8) You will sometimes be asked questions that your partner would like to be asked by you in return. "Did that scene work for you?" he asks. "Yes, did you like it too?" Then his answer, "Well yes, I liked it lots, but there's one thing that made a problem for me...and I am afraid to talk about it because I don't know how you will react..."

9) These conversations will usually be initiated by the person who is the most comfortable with the process. He must remember that it might not be so easy for the other one.

10) Don't expect instant answers. Some of us must take our time to figure out just how it is that we feel about something before we can talk about it. Also, just because he can talk comfortably about piss trips, do not assume it will be equally easy for him to talk about pain trips.

11) Try to be complete with your questions, answers and comments. Take your time, and think about it before you answer. These are important conversations. Try to give your serious attention to the discussion, to each other, and to yourself.

"Yes, I would like a piercing, and it scares me a lot." "Yes, the scene was great, and I wish it had been longer." "No, I did not want you to lick my boots, because at the bar, some guy at the urinal missed, and hit them instead. I did not want you to lick some stranger's piss off my boots because I don't think that is safe to do anymore." "Well, I know part of the answer to your question, but not all. Let me think about it a few days, and I'll let you know what I come up with."

12) It is critical that any issues about safety be discussed at these times. Remember, consciousness about safety is not

universal yet. So you might get comments like these: "It is impossible for me to surrender to some scene when I am unsure about the cleanliness of the equipment. Will it be OK if I clean such and such myself in the future?" Or, "I was afraid when you wanted to use the whatsit that Richard gave you last week, because I saw blood on it then. And you didn't say whether you had cleaned it yet or not. That's why I backed away from you when I did. I don't want to catch hepatitis or AIDS from somebody's toy."

Or, "You really must tell me when your wrists are going to sleep in the future, because I don't want to have to deal with nerve damage, and I want you to be able to cook dinner for me!" Or, "I get scared when you whip me that hard with the heavy whip, because I worry about a cracked rib or something. Where can we find out about my concern?" Or, "From now on, I will feel safer about putting you in a hood if you will promise me to use a decongestant inhaler to clear your sinuses first, so there's less chance of you developing a breathing problem like you did last night."

13) Support your partner by telling him why you like the way he plays. Reread suggestion #4.

If you want the words to come out just right about a touchy subject, don't hesitate to rehearse things when you are alone in the car or in the bathroom. Try to think how you would feel if he said the same things to you, and adjust the words accordingly till it says just what you really mean. Work hard with your language to remove criticism—your partner needs your support to change his behavior, not your hostility.

Use this baker's dozen of suggestions in your efforts to get talking about your scenes with your partner. Take some time to really think about what you have said and what you have heard after these conversations, so that you can learn from them. Thank each other for the information. After all, you need it to get closer to where you want to go. If you love him, don't forget to tell him so.

During the scene

It is time to start talking about how you communicate with your partner as the scene is unfolding. My hope is that you can think about how some of these ideas might apply to your own playing style and perhaps enhance your experiences in scenes.

Let's begin with the element of time. It's important to note that a "scene" will often begin before the "action" part starts to happen. Likewise, the "scene" usually does not end until what I call "re-entry" into standard day-to-day mood has been smoothly accomplished. These are generalizations, of course, and there are fine scenes happening that lack the pre-action and post-action phases.

My point in mentioning all this is that movement through these phases is usually accompanied by changes in the communication style of the players. One handy way to think of a scene is to think of the five speed transmissions found in fine cars. First gear only takes you so fast. To go faster (farther) you need to leave first gear behind and shift up to second and so on. Likewise, you may start in "first gear" when you meet someone in a bar, at a party, or wherever. As you cruise and become interested, and begin to detect mutual interest, you might want to think about escalating the intensity of your exchange by shifting into "second gear," so to speak. For many guys nowadays, this shift is usually into a conversation about safer sex issues. It can include any other negotiations about the content of the hoped for scene.

If there is agreement about safer sex matters, and you think there might be an SM fit, a shift to "third gear" might then happen. This could include more intimate touching, moving a bit closer during conversation, less talk and more looking, dealing with logistics like, "can we do this tonight, and where," and "do you have a car parked somewhere?" In this gear, we can ask essential questions like, "do you have to work tomorrow?" and "have you taken drugs of any kind?" And we can start setting the scene with queries like, "can we make noise at your place?" You know the stuff I mean.

162

Importantly, this communication "gear" can, and often does include some hot talk which may or may not hint at possibilities for the anticipated "action." In fact, at this point, the action portion of the scene may have already begun in the minds of one or both players. "I have a hot little room that I'd like to see you strung up in for a few hours or so." Or, "I would really be glad for the chance to try to be of some service to you, Sir."

So far, I have been describing a typical connection between strangers meeting for the first or second time. Moving through the first and second communication "gears" can take five minutes or five weeks. If you are already in a relationship, you will usually start your movement toward a scene with "third gear" type communications. This will sound different than between strangers. So you might get, "I am hoping for some hot time with you on Saturday night, because something very special came in the mail yesterday that I want to introduce you to..." Or, "Yes, I will enjoy going out for a while, but I want to save enough time tonight to play with you, so wear something that will make my dick hard, and get on you knees when we get home." Or, "I spent some time polishing your boots earlier and got a hardon. Is there something I can do to make you feel...better?"

In "fourth gear," the beginning of the action portion of the scene, typically (yes, of course there are exceptions aplenty) the Top, *if He is the dominant sort*, tends to determine the amount, variety, and direction of the verbal (with words) communications. The bottom, *if he is the submissive sort*, tends to determine the amount and variety of non-verbal communication (sounds that are not words, and movements of both body and eyes).

For example, in scenes that I have had the honor to watch between dominant Tops and submissive bottoms, the bottoms quite often do not speak except to use safe words if available, to answer the Top's questions, and to make reports about body conditions. A bottom might say, for example, "I think I should tell you that I'm getting cold," or, "The knots on the left side are slipping." "My contact lenses are still in", or, "Sir, my hands are falling asleep and will be completely asleep in about 10 minutes or so."

Conversely, bottoms tend to respond to whatever the Top is doing with a wide range of sounds and movements that reveal their reactions to whatever is happening. In general, Tops do more talking in a scene than bottoms, and bottoms make more wordless sound. In many SM relationships that have stabilized, the men will often play together for hours with scarcely any words exchanged whatsoever. That doesn't mean they aren't communicating. They just don't feel the need to use many words.

Many bottoms who consider themselves to be successful players have told me, both in and out of the therapy room, that they tend to prefer to communicate with Tops in non-verbal ways during the "action" part of the scene. If an important problem develops, they are more willing to use words.

Some skilled bottoms can purposely inform Tops about the tightness of restraints merely by glancing at a tight one with a frown or with an accompanying twisting motion in the wrist. I know of bottoms who have stopped unsuccessful scenes cold just by faking something having gotten in their eye. They can encourage a Top to whip them harder (or softer) just by moving their ass or back a bit differently, or with a smile or a groan of pleasure. All this, and more, without words of any sort.

In the past, I have often spoken and written about "cuing." These non-verbal communications are just other examples of the art of cuing at work. Of course, bottom cues are wasted on Tops who don't know how to read them and those who miss them altogether! Obviously, there are also Tops who have no interest in a bottom's cues. They will do exactly as they please up to, and in some cases, beyond the bottom's limits.

My guess about all this is that by choosing not to use words unless it's urgent, these bottoms reinforce the feeling in the scene that the Top is in total charge of events. They do this because they believe it makes their scenes hotter. This can support a Top in a scene and encourage him to be more spontaneous. In actuality, for scenes with these bottoms, events in the scene are influenced by both Top and bottom.

Fifth gear happens when the players fall into a comfort with each other that allows them to feel that the scene is going to work out well. The communication exchanges are smooth and complete enough to get the job done without being excessive. Things are hot, and it's happening. At this point, they can kick the scene into neutral whenever they want a rest, and go right back into high gear again.

When the action portion of the scene seems over, the "re-entry" portion of the scene begins. Some guys refer to this as the "coming down" part. If the scene has gone well, the partners are usually in a non-drug "high" (also called an "SM high" by some) and are feeling very close to each other and to themselves. This "high," which is an altered state of consciousness, is a desirable state for most folks in the scene, and is the usual payoff for doing SM in the first place.

The SM "High" can be sustained for quite some time, depending on how the re-entry is managed. If the bottom is really wiped out at this point, the management of these moments is usually in the hands of Top. Often, good SM between guys in a relationship creates a sort of hypnotic spell between them when the scene ends. This "spell" will be broken if five minutes later one of the guys starts talking about work or something unrelated to the emotional setting that has just been created by playing.

The altered state of consciousness that I refer to here is threatening for some people. So is the intimacy that goes with it. If this kind of intense intimacy is scary for one of the players, he may try to break the "spell" of the SM High as soon as possible by talking about something unrelated to what is happening in the room, or by immediately starting to fuss with his clothes or start cleaning up. He will do anything to escape the intimacy.

Disturbing the SM High during the re-entry can make for a rough landing emotionally for the other player. When either one breaks the spell, the other often feels discarded, abandoned, foolish, or unappreciated. When the spell is broken by one, the other often reports the feeling that he has just been used like a court jester for the other's amusement. This can hurt.

These reentry times are moments to be cherished and lingered over like fine wine or a favorite painting, or perhaps a special sunset. These are times for touching and the little tendernesses that say how you feel about sharing this time in your lives. These are the moments in which SM becomes part of the glue that holds your relationship together and makes it so special. Please don't rush past—you will miss something wonderful that is found nowhere else.

Who's Running This Show, Anyway?

"Consistency is the last refuge of the unimaginative."

—Oscar Wilde

For a long time now, I have heard the question come up in conversations, "Who is in control of a scene, the Top or the bottom?" I assume that this question is important because folks wonder if they are "doing it right," or if their partner is "doing it right." I have finally realized that there are five answers to this question: In some scenes, the person in charge is the Top; in others, it is the bottom; in others, both; in others, neither the Top nor the bottom is in control; and in yet others, the control passes back and forth.

Let me explain. In scenes between very dominant Tops and very submissive bottoms, the balance of power is most often tipped in favor of the Top. But some kinds of Tops are very submissive (I know several very passive sadists, for example), and they prefer to play with rather dominant bottoms. In these scenes, the balance of power is most often tipped in favor of the bottom, and everybody seems happy.

In scenes between sadist and masochist where neither is dominant or submissive, both may share in the control of the scene about equally, and that is usually satisfactory. In other sorts of scenes, especially those where drug use is a prominent feature, it seems as though neither player is in charge (maybe the drugs are in charge—spooky to contemplate). In scenes between men who switch back and forth, the control element in the scene may pass back and forth between the players comfortably.

This is worth mentioning here because the power

configurations in a scene can often determine the communication style that works for the players. For example, some bottoms like to take a strong role in the direction of a scene.

Those bottoms who are into penetration scenes—especially fisting, but also catheters, dildoes, piercing, and some whipping as well as plain ole fucking—will often feel that taking a strong role is the only way they can really protect themselves from the possibility of viral contamination or injury. They will have a better time if they choose Tops who like to be taught, or ones who are rather passive with their sadism. Such Tops exist, and they prefer bottoms who send very clear signals about their needs. A Top of this type is relieved at not having to make up a scene for the bottom to enjoy. He doesn't have to risk the rejection that he feels goes with trying something the bottom might not like.

On the other hand, submissive bottoms get frustrated with passive Tops who don't want to *take charge* of a scene. These bottoms will do better to spend their time with dominant Tops, who will be more than happy to take charge of a scene. Dominant Tops complain long and loud about "pushy" bottoms, because these Tops often feel ripped off when dealing with dominant/pushy bottoms. I have come to believe that this complaining results either when a bottom has misled a Top during their initial come-on to each other, or the Top thought he could break a pushy bottom into a submissive one, and failed.

There is a place in this world for "pushy" type bottoms, just as there is a place in this world for passive Tops. The time spent by dominant Tops complaining about "pushy" bottoms would be better spent in looking for a quality submissive instead.

I do not mean to suggest that Tops only have one style for all occasions. They don't, and neither do bottoms. How we are going to approach our counterparts is often determined by what mood we are in at the time. In the vast majority of us, there are several very different kinds of Tops, and several different sorts of bottoms too. Just stop to think about how many different ways you, yourself have played, *and* achieved satisfaction, and you will see my point.

For example, a bottom may be more assertive if he is out looking for some sort of more risky penetration scene, whereas he may be much more submissive if he is feeling the need to serve as a boot slave for the evening. Likewise, a Top who is out looking for his favorite scene, something at which he is very accomplished and confident, is likely to approach a bottom in a very dominant way. At other times, the same guy might want to learn about something new, like electricity for example, and go for the bottom who can step him through the scene, wire by wire, so to speak. In short, there may be many different, comfortable ways for a Top to be a Top—same for bottoms.

Every day is a new day, and we can get into trouble when we expect ourselves to be the same person in the bar this weekend as we were last weekend. In the same way, it is unwise to assume that just because we observe someone in an aggressive style one week that he is going to be that way next week also. Maybe Mother was right when she suggested that I try to take people at face value.

The issue of "who is in control" is much less important than the issue of "are you getting your needs met in the scene." This has to be the bottom line or else, what's the point?

Tops: Out In The Cold?

The squeakiest wheel gets the grease.

—American proverb

For some time now, the information available about the SM/leather scene, especially from a technical point of view, has been dominated by a forest of safety information designed primarily to protect bottoms from physical and psychological injury at the hand of inept, inexperienced or indifferent Tops. This preoccupation with safety concerns has had several results: 1) Many bottoms have begun to feel safer when they play, even with strangers. More bottoms have gotten more involved at deeper levels in the scene, and the scene has opened up some. 2) Tops and bottoms have become more technically proficient, and more willing to undertake more technically demanding (and risky) scenes. 3) It *seems* that there are fewer unintentional SM injuries than happened, say in 1973. (Breath control play remains the most likely way to get into terminal trouble in a scene.) 4) Novices (both Tops & bottoms) can become technically proficient much faster than was possible even a few years ago. 5) The dissemination of technical information has given the SM clubs a focal point for outreach and network-building in the community.

Certainly, there have been other benefits to this preoccupation with safety concerns as well, but there has been at least one important downside to this, and it has largely been ignored. *What about Top's needs?*

In the rush to make the world safe for bottoms, Tops have been forgotten about, partly because the risk of physical, which is to say, *obvious* injury, has distracted most of us from the "other half" of the SM equation. Unfortunately, Tops have

171

come to be seen as the ones to watch out for—the loose cannons on the ship's deck. All the preoccupations with bottom's needs for safety have had the effect of psychologically bludgeoning Tops into believing that they must become technical wizards, or risk getting terrible reputations in their respective communities. This is sad because Tops get little enough support as is.

Tops have told me that they have felt psychologically castrated by the bottom-centered values that became dominant in the SM scene in the late '80s. Castrated Tops are not happy Tops, and some have just plain given up on the likelihood of having a good ol' rip-roarin' time working some guy over, and putting him through his paces.

It is true that a Top must be technically competent enough to avoid unwanted injuries and protect himself and his partners from disease. But it is also true that the SM encounter must be a hard-on for a Top once he has dealt with the safety issues. Otherwise, he will look for other ways to have a good time. One Top friend mentioned to me that he was having a better time at the Country/Western bars these days because the leather bars had stopped being the friendly places that they once were in some cities.

It is unclear just how this situation has come about. I suspect it is related to the fact that it is much easier for bottoms to talk about what does not work for them than it is for Tops to talk about what does work for them. Consequently, we have a lot more information about what bottoms need from a scene than we have about what Tops need from the same encounter. In fact, many Tops have a hard time talking about what they like about SM, even in the therapy room. Being a Top, it seems, is a more private experience than being a bottom.

Even in friendly conversation with Tops, it can take a while to learn that they are interested in more than the bottom's good time. Some like to witness suffering of their own creation. Others are into controlling another person. Still others are terrorists who like to scare or threaten bottoms. There are those Tops who are thrilled to demean or humiliate their partner.

Arrogant Tops will sometimes enjoy ignoring or prick-teasing the bottoms they play with. Some Tops like to be worshiped as demi-gods. Yet others seek only the reputations that go with becoming skilled technicians. The idea of using another man as a personal sexual toy is the turn on for most sorts of Tops in general. Depersonalization is what gets other Tops off. The range is not endless, but it is vast, and may shift from day to day or year to year.

In our society, like it or not, being dominant and/or sadistic is unfortunately (my opinion now) associated with self-sufficiency and independence, privacy, and, above all, with big-M masculinity. Conversely, being submissive and/or masochistic is also associated with dependency, neediness, letting feelings show, vulnerability, and with big-F femininity.

Given the pull of these stereotypes, who can be surprised that we have more information about the needs of bottoms than the needs of Tops. According to the masculine stereotype, a Top is supposed to be self-contained. In the SM scene, that translates to isolated—maybe even from himself!

Many hours in the therapy room have led me to the conclusion that the association of masculinity, dominance and being self-contained has fostered the mistaken impression in many Tops' minds that they don't need bottoms, even that needing bottoms is an admission of weakness. For some, it feels like it is even a character flaw.

From my point of view, Tops and bottoms must form erotic teams. Without our respective counterparts, we are frustrated, and cannot get our rather exotic needs met. It seems that we do need each other to create the kind of experiences that we desire, and in which we find a special kind of fulfillment. It is clear to me that our (yes, both Tops' and bottoms') enemy is our unconscious allegiance to a screwed up masculine stereotype that doesn't work any better for us gay leathermen than it does for straight men or women.

Those with dominant and/or sadistic needs must find a way to free themselves of the need to appear self-contained, and they must start to talk about what they really *need* to *feel* and *do* in a scene with a hot bottom. Until these things happen, the SM scene will continue to be bottom-focused, simply because bottoms can talk better about what they need out of a scene.

What can be done about all this? Here are some suggestions that I hope can start the process of encouraging the tribe to support Tops as well as it has begun to support bottoms.

1) You Tops can begin the process in the privacy of your very own bedroom if you like, just by spending some quiet time with yourselves thinking about what you want for yourselves from an SM encounter. If you can feel safe about doing so, keep a journal of some sort in which you tell yourself the truth about what you want. Remember to protect any such writings from the eyes of outsiders.

2) Those local organizations with SM as their focus could consider instituting an ongoing discussion group for Tops and switches, the purpose of which would be to provide a forum for people to share honestly their thoughts and feelings about what the SM encounter holds for them as Tops. Try not to allow these meetings to become a setting in which Tops try to out do each other with hot stories about past exploits.

3) The writers (both fiction and non-fiction) and other artists among us can start to produce a more emotionally balanced exploration of the dominant/sadistic mind set. We need more good poetry, and Tops need to read it. Reading poetry is also a masculine pursuit. Remember the Samurai warrior!

4) National organizations can consider offering workshops and other sorts of presentations that move toward offering better definition and clarity to the dominant/sadistic experience.

Most importantly, Tops can start talking with themselves, with each other, and with bottoms about their needs in honest ways. It will be out of these conversations that a more balanced set of values can grow, and our tribe's *preoccupation* with bottom values will be ended.

The Trouble With Tops

"There's nothing worse than a Top who
won't deal with reality."

—Mr. Bannon

Many times clients have come in complaining about a Top they met over the weekend, and what a lousy time was had by all. My plan here is to recount some of the more common themes about Top behavior that cause bottoms to despair of finding a satisfying relationship.

In the next essay, I share some of my thoughts about "Killer Bottoms," and the ways they can derail Tops and make relationships tough. First, though, we'll look at what I've learned from my work with their counterparts, "Killer" Tops. They, too, can be equally responsible when relationships either don't get off the ground, or crash and burn. Tops need to have positive reinforcing experiences with bottoms, or they will turn sour on the scene. The same holds true for bottoms: Listen up, Tops!

Bottom complaints about Tops tend to come to me mostly in two forms; technical incompetence, and person-to-person incompetence. These days, there is so much technical information available about how to do almost anything in the realm of SM, that it is astonishing to me that the technical sort of complaints are still happening. Fortunately, there are numerous clubs, publications, and videos available, many of which go into the most minute details about how to do everything from handling a 10 foot bullwhip to elaborate piercings and bondage set ups. Some organizations have phone numbers available with which callers can get the most obscure sorts of technical information while remaining completely anonymous, if that is the caller's wish.

In fact, technical information is so available now, that when I hear about technical errors in a scene, I often suspect that maybe the Top didn't want the information in the first place! At best, perhaps the Top couldn't let himself get the needed training. Ask yourself, "why wouldn't a Top want as much technical information as possible, going into a scene?"

Well, some Tops feel humiliated or embarrassed to admit that there might be something that they don't already know about, and aren't expert at doing. In this sense, these Tops are just like other people who have trouble asking for what they need. However, in the SM scene, that can lead to trouble.

The most common "diagnosis" for these Tops is: Superman complex and fragile ego. These are people who expect themselves to know everything and to do everything perfectly the first time. This is really a people-to-people problem masquerading as a technical problem. In general, relationship problems can be expected when one partner believes that he knows everything about anything. I have yet to meet anyone who knows all about SM.

It is important to note that even the most experienced person can have accidents while doing a scene. "Shit happens." Sometimes, a Killer Bottom may be at work in these situations. Such bottoms sometimes like to seduce unwary Tops into playing beyond their skill levels—accidents are almost guaranteed. But usually, the responsibility for accidents lies with the Top, who, at least ritualistically, needs to be in charge of what goes on in a scene. Accidents in scenes between mutualists (players who are both Top and bottom at the same time) may be the responsibility of either player or both, but I digress.

Bottom complaints about Top person-to-person skills tend to be much more frequent and strident. I have come to believe that a bottom is much more likely to be wounded emotionally than physically.

Most dangerous are the Tops who play from an angry place. They somehow get the idea that bottoms are people whose lot

176

in life is to be punching bags for Tops who have had a bad day at the office or a rough time on the freeway. Even worse are the guys who just plain have angry personalities. They go looking for somebody who really wants to get beat up. But, quite often, they run into a bottom who simply wants a plain old heavy scene, and mistake him for their hoped-for "victim." The results are sometimes not pretty, and most often not fun for the bottom.

I have seen it time and again in my practice: when people play from anger, limits often are not respected, and consent vanishes. The Top can become a rapist. Not many bottoms who have experienced real rape go back for more. Few bottoms object to being used consensually; most object to being systematically abused. There is a big difference. Satisfying relationships are usually not possible with abusers of any stripe.

From a technical point of view, Tops who play from their anger tend to make mistakes when they play, because anger makes people hurry—they play faster than they can think responsibly. Most experienced players know that good SM doesn't mix well with speed (of any kind). As bottoms become experienced, they tend to figure this out and usually start avoiding the Tops who feel angry and deliver their scenes rapidfire fast.

More confusing to bottoms are the Tops who have internal conflicts about their need to dominate and/or about their sadism. They can get distant the next day, even after a good scene. Some need one too many drinks in them before they can ever play, or must always take drugs to get into it. Tops with this trouble will sometimes become switches, transiting to the bottom side to "work off" guilty feelings about having dominated someone or played heavily with a bottom. Others drive (punish?) themselves extra hard at work to re-balance.

Usually, this is all unconscious, and the Top doesn't know it's happening until weirdness with relationships brings him into therapy. Once the guilty feelings about the need to dominate get resolved, the Top will be more able to enter relationships, without feeling guilty every time he plays with his bottom.

177

Sometimes, a Top who wants out of a relationship, or even a new courtship, will drive the bottom away by increasing the severity of the scenes, exceeding capabilities, until the bottom cracks and bails out of the relationship first. The fleeing bottom goes away feeling inadequate when the real problem was that the Top couldn't initiate an honest and straightforward conversation. How could such a Top hope to establish a satisfying relationship until he learns to talk honestly?

Other Tops run into trouble when they go into a scene with a particular agenda. Sometimes they have a standard play sequence: First, I'll tie him up, then some tit scenes, then a condom fuck, followed by some rigid bondage, blah, blah, blah.... It never occurs to these Tops that perhaps their very practiced delivery might feel mechanical or rehearsed to the bottom. With this kind of Top, bottom soon feels that maybe just any ol' bottom would do, and there is nothing personal about the scene. This is an instant turn off (except maybe for the novices). Everyone likes to feel special.

Many Tops never figure out that most bottoms will surrender themselves more completely and more quickly when they are made to feel special. Tops who want relationships will be more successful if they know when to "try a little tenderness," even (especially?!) during a scene.

Deeply satisfying relationships are things that happen between people who are emotionally complete with each other. This completeness is possible when a person has access to the total range of emotions with which to respond to the world and the events in it. In fact, some systems of psychotherapy define mental un-wellness in terms of narrowness of emotional range. When certain feelings are banished from our repertoire, we become diminished as people. Those Tops who always present themselves as hot erotic drawings often leave bottoms who thirst for relationships wondering if there is a real live person in there somewhere.

When I see ads requiring that bottoms be "young," I often suspect that these Tops may be unable to deal with experienced bottoms who make more emotional demands than novices.

Young bottoms are much less likely than guys who have been around the track before to call Tops on their shit, or the mistreatment they give bottoms. Most young guys don't know any better, and are willing to settle for less than emotional completeness. This strategy takes the pressure off Tops to be real, but often makes for short, flat and stormy relationships that can be downright dangerous.

Tops with nothing but attitude may work fine for a scene or two, but where are they when a friend dies and you need a shoulder? What can you expect of them when you are sick and don't want to be alone when you have to throw up? Sometimes intimacy is extra-demanding, and at those times, a real person is called for; two dimensional Tops just will not do. The SM relationships I have seen working out well work best when all partners can move easily back and forth between the complex realities of daily living and the erotic requirements of our scene.

I recall, a long time ago, reading a Heinlein story about a fellow named Lazarus Long who defined a man (this part is foggy) as someone who could plan a battle, set a broken leg, arrange flowers, dance 'till dawn, shoot to kill, cook a good meal.... I don't recall exactly all the attributes, but Heinlein's sense of it was that a real man is not a tightass. Some academic commentators have noted that homosexual life has become so "virilized" that our idealized subculture heros are just laughable caricatures of stereotyped masculinity. I am sure that, in many cases, they are correct. Leather bars are loaded with stereotypes.

Yet, it is also true that stereotypes can be fun to play with and otherwise enjoy. At the same time, my work has forced me to conclude that stereotypical manhood *all by itself* ain't so great when it comes to forging durable and satisfying relationships. Ask almost any straight woman.

My best advice to those Tops looking for relationships is to learn when to get *real*, and when to get *hot*, and how to be comfortable with both. My best advice to bottoms is not to settle for less.

Beware The Killer Bottom

In lectures and articles, I have urged people to see the importance of doing SM relationships "your own way," without the undue influence of porno stereotypes or peer pressure. This should not be taken to mean that it's OK to abandon the principles of safe, sane, and consensual.

Usually, we tend to think about these words in terms of responsibilities that belong to the Top in a scene or a relationship. They apply equally to bottoms, in ways you may not have thought about yet. I refer to interpersonal safety, sanity, and consensuality. What do I mean?

In the therapy room, I have worked with many Tops who have been mauled emotionally by bottoms, both in one-night scenes, and in ongoing relationships. There had been no consent given. The stereotypes would have us believe that Tops have all the power to harm, and that bottoms are just helpless bundles of vulnerability. Nonsense.

Bottoms have lots of power too, and they are in danger of harming when they don't know it, don't acknowledge it, don't want it, or don't respect it. A friend once referred to bottoms who don't properly recognize and respond to their own power as "Killer Bottoms," and I think maybe it fits.

Example: Non-submission, or "Please, Sir, I'll wear whatever you pick out for me." In this scenario, the Top chooses clothing for his bottom, then catches a frown of disapproval. The bottom hoped his Top would mind-read, and pick something else for the occasion. In this example, the bottom uses his power in a destructive way by first offering submission, then criticizing the form of the Top's dominance. A more creative use of power might have been for this bottom to have assessed the Top's taste in clothing and style before offering this particular submission.

Another example: Criticism. Top ties bottom up with rope, and bottom responds with, "I can tell you have never done this before." Or, "You did it so much better last month." Presto! Bottom has either created an angry Top, or he has hurt a Top's feelings. Yes, Tops have feelings.

Guess what bottoms! Tops with hurt feelings won't want to do it again, and might mention to others that you don't have good scene manners. Angry Tops can get more nasty than you can imagine, or throw you out, or bad mouth you, or ignore you—none of which is probably what you wanted in the first place.

The power to criticize is also the power to inform or seduce. The same bottom in the above situation might have more creatively used this power: "This is new. I've never had anyone tie me so loosely before." Or, "May I report such and such about my wrists?" Or, how about this: "Say, Mister, I wonder if there might be some service I could perform that would persuade you to make those tighter (looser)." Lastly, the bottom might say nothing, but move his body in such a way so as to reveal that the bondage just doesn't work. None of these responses judges the Top, and all of them support the scene continuing.

One thing I have clearly noticed is that budding Tops, as a group, seem less willing to tolerate disappointing initial experiences than do new bottoms. Tops just coming into the scene will need to have positive initial experiences with bottoms, or else they will try to get their sadistic/dominant needs met elsewhere—probably through work.

This observation may account for the fact that the ratio of Tops to bottoms is so lopsided. The irony, if I am right about this, is that Killer Bottoms may themselves be responsible for the smaller number of Tops in the scene. It may be that the egos of only the most durable Tops can survive the coming out process.

There are other varieties of Killer bottoms. One sort is the "bottomless bottom." These are the ones who can never be satisfied no matter how long or how hard they are played.

(Drugs?) Tops often report feeling burned out after playing with them, and come to prefer bottoms who can be fulfilled in a scene.

Another type is the bottom who is so controlling in the scene that Tops begin to suspect they are dealing with a Top in bottom drag. Some Tops like the adversarial quality of these encounters, but most Tops seem to come away from them feeling topped by the bottom. This often depresses Tops, leaving them feeling like they've been "had" in some way.

Sometimes, one of these bottoms gets hold of a novice Top. New Tops, not yet knowing how to negotiate scenes with these "Toppy" bottoms, can later discover that they feel castrated and foolish. This is trial by fire for novice Tops, and some do not survive.

An irony here is that when bottoms try to control too much in a scene, the Top's creativity and spontaneity can suffer almost total destruction. Bottom then gets his wish, an opportunity to complain about the Top's abilities.

Obviously, I have talked to many Tops who have complaints about bottoms. Not surprisingly, I have also spent hours talking to Killer Bottoms. It is clear to me that only a few bottoms ever set out to become the Killer type. So, how does it happen? I have come to believe that the Killer Bottom syndrome develops in one of two main ways.

First, some bottoms have very negative attitudes about submission and surrender, even though they feel drawn to them. This sets up a war within the self which expresses itself in ambivalent feelings. They send Tops double messages (I want to submit—I won't submit—You will submit).

Secondly, other bottoms both fear and hope that Tops will hurt or engulf them. These bottoms send both seductive and defensive signals to Tops. Tops see them as prick teasers, or read their communications as "I'm not ready yet" messages. Tops burn out fast with this type.

Implied in all this discussion is something that no one talks about much, and that is that Tops can be fragile too. Bottoms don't like to look at this idea because "it don't much fit their fantasies." Many bottoms dream of Tops who are made of steel, and feel nothing. For many bottoms, its tough to think about surrendering to someone whom they could hurt. That's more responsibility than they want, or know how to deal with.

Tops need selective reinforcement from bottoms if they are to remain in the scene and flourish. Maybe, just maybe, certain bottom behaviors are themselves the reason for the lopsided Top to bottom distribution in the scene. Perhaps bottoms, by modifying their behavior with some of these ideas in mind, could change that.

I am not saying that Killer Bottoms are doing it wrong, but I don't have the impression that their style works well for either bottoms or Tops. Of course, everyone has the right to persist in behaviors that don't work.

I know there are bad Tops out there, but when bottoms complain about the scene, I have to wonder where the problem really is. Everyone must take responsibility for the quality of the lifestyle or it won't improve. This means bottoms as well as Tops.

Thinking About Consent

*"If you beat the shit out of a man, he will
learn all about you."*

—Nigel Kent

In my thinking, the word relationship stands for a large
idea. For me, even during the briefest encounter with a waitress
or salesclerk, a relationship happens. These short relationships
have the capacity to be satisfying exchanges if we keep our
heads screwed on straight about things. Excepting the genetic
relationship we have with our families of origin and
relationships with the authorities, all other relationships require
some degree of consent. Certainly, for any relationship to
develop and/or become more intimate, mutual consent is an
absolute requirement. This includes our relationships with our
Selves.

Normally, the ability to give one's consent begins to appear
in early childhood, matures in teenage years, and is refined in
adulthood. It then lasts until senility, illness or death strips it
from us. Involuntary torture or imprisonment, drug addiction,
brainwashing and hypnosis all raise special issues,
but for most of us, consent is an everyday part of our lives.

When we come to an SM encounter, the workings of
consent are useful to understand, because *not* understanding
them can produce an unsatisfying scene, unwanted injury or
worse. It can mean the difference between staying in the scene
or bailing out.

How does consent work? Well, some part of our mind is
always paying attention to what is happening, and making
constant evaluations about the action and the interaction with
our partner(s). It is a bit like having a traffic signal in our heads

with green, yellow and red lights.

In the age of safer sex practices, we have all had to become even more aware about this "traffic light," and pay attention to the information we get from it. Most SM/leather folks have known about this "light" all along, because we have had to use it to make scenes work better for us long before serious health concerns came into play.

Basically, the "traffic light" in our mind works by testing the action with questions like these: is it safe, does this feel "good," is it what I want to be happening, is it what I need, is it what he needs, what would father think, will I respect myself/him in the morning, is this sinful, and perhaps many others as well. The "light" is always on, shining red, yellow, and green whenever we are awake.

To achieve satisfaction from the SM experience, a person must be able to consult this inner "traffic light," and be able to read and respond to its information appropriately.

For example, if things are working fine in the scene (green light), and suddenly something happens—the bottom starts to look faint or disoriented, the Top looks like he might be getting into position to fuck without a rubber, the bottom begins to react for no apparent reason, the Top goes over and picks up a toy that is scary or dangerous—*then* the consent "light" may change to yellow or even red. What happens is that our consent comfort is diminished, at least temporarily.

One or the other partner will usually do or say something about the change. Following the above examples, Top might say, "You look faint or something, are you alright?" His light has also turned yellow now, and he wants to suspend his consent to continue until he satisfies himself that bottom is in condition to continue.

The bottom who fears the Top may try an unprotected fuck feels his light turn yellow, and might say, "Fucking without a rubber won't work for me anymore, Sir," or, "A fuck is a good idea, but I'll need some conversation about it first, please." The bottom here is saying that he won't continue without a change in the Top's behavior, one which will turn his lights green

186

again. Top, in this situation, can reassure bottom just by saying something like, "I just want to look at the merchandise for now."

The Top, seeing or hearing some unexpected reaction, might feel his light turn yellow, and say, "What's going on with you?" The bottom's reaction may have broken their connection, and the Top wants to reconnect before he will be willing to continue. If he is unsuccessful, the light will turn red, and the scene will stop, at least for a time.

Or, seeing the Top go for a piece of equipment that is too scary, a bottom might report the change in his light color by saying, "The worst scene I ever had was with one of those, and they make me nervous as hell." Or even, "If we are going to continue, I need some more conversation about that thing first, please."

My point here is that consent is a moment-by-moment gift that the players in a scene give to each other and can take away at will. This is most especially true the first time you play with someone—even the first few times. "Consent" means that any player has the ability to influence (but not necessarily control) the pace and intensity of an encounter, and may end it at will, or say "No" in the first place. Modern day players, exploring the sexual frontier, would do well to avoid anyone who does not, or will not subscribe to this idea in advance.

Occasionally, I run across a top (small t intentional here!) who approaches bottoms with an attitude of "once you have submitted to me, you are mine to do with as I choose, and you like it or lump it." One such that I know of in Los Angeles is forever complaining (sometimes in print) about how frustrated he is in his quest to find slaves. He runs ads for them rather regularly it seems. Most Tops have discovered that they can't order consent as if it were just a Pizza with sausage and bell pepper. It seems that he wants them to give their consent, then the "slave" gets to deal with the consequences, come what may. This top will most likely end up with fools or novices for slaves—how sad for all concerned. How meaningful could such total and instantaneous consent really be?

My personal view is that any candidate slave or bottom who would accept such "all or nothing" terms going into a scene is flirting with disaster. I, myself, accepted such terms once and was in the emergency room three hours later. I had chosen to ignore the information I was getting from my internal "traffic signal." It was a costly lesson, one I vowed never to repeat.

Yet, I did have to learn it all over again as a Top. I have been equally mauled (emotionally) by castrating and manipulative bottoms when I chose to ignore the warnings of my own Top "traffic signal." I should have redirected the scene when the first yellow warnings registered on my consciousness. We live, and hopefully, we learn.

If people respond quickly and clearly to the yellow signal when it happens, then the lights (ideally) will never get to the red stage unless an accident occurs, or until everybody is played out.

As we get more practice playing with the same person, perhaps a regular kinky fuck buddy, the consent gift becomes cautiously extended. For example, as a bottom, suppose I know from previous scenes that a particular play partner is a tit specialist, and he initiates a tit scene of some sort. I am more willing to cut him some slack than if I suddenly see him reach for a bullwhip, something I have never seen him use that I know can be dangerous in the wrong hands. Or, as a Top, suppose I have played a lot whipping some special whip lover, and he has come to trust me. One day I decide to indulge a wish for rigid bondage. My own light turns yellow automatically because I know that the requirements of the two scenes are very different. My consent will be very cautious until I learn whether, and how well, he can tolerate the scene.

It is unwise to assume that consent in one area of technique will carry over into another quite different technical area.

As we get more and more experience with the same person or group of people, the consent gift lengthens in time. Consent may be given for an entire evening. Sometimes an agreement not to try anything new may set everyone's mind more at ease, and keep the "traffic light" glowing green for the whole evening.

For those who become involved in ongoing relationships where SM is part of the understood sexuality, partners may come to a place where the consent is unreserved, given until further notice. Partners sometimes present themselves for counseling when something has happened in a scene where one or both partners felt their consent was violated in some way.

Most men I know with SM relationships take their sexuality seriously. As a result, there can be major fallout when the consent stuff breaks down. It can threaten the relationship entirely if there is no mending.

As you may have guessed, the giving of consent is closely related to the development of trust as the scene unfolds. As trust increases, consent is the likely outcome. Conversely, as the trust decreases—and it can vanish in an instant—the consent drops off sharply. All this requires players to pay attention to their feelings during a scene. This is how we get information from our internal "traffic signals." As always, drugs, including alcohol of course, make accurate reading of our feelings more difficult, more so as we consume more of whatever.

My advice to newcomers to the SM scene is to try to keep your consent levels equal to your feelings of trust. If you are a bottom and are slow to trust Tops, then so be it. Not all Tops are for you, but some Tops love to slowly get inside your head, and gradually develop your trust. This way, your consent and submission means more to them—it is an achievement. They feel all the better for the conquest.

If you are a novice Top and are slow to trust, so be it. Wary bottoms may not work well for you—the more experienced men who are less threatened by dominance may be a better bet. Interview!

Consent is one of the cornerstones of modern day Leather/SM morality. Without it, we run the risk of becoming the rapists that the rest of society assumes us to be. Among other things, SM is a highly-styled and carefully-managed vulnerability for both Top and bottom. Without the requirement of consent, an SM scene runs the risk of going out of control, crossing the line into assault. Today, there is no more room in the SM scene for sexual anarchists—they have already caused us too much trouble. Understanding just how consent works will defend you from them whether they are Tops or bottoms.

Pushing Limits:
When Consent Can Get
In The Way...

In the last seven years or so, it has become common and somewhat fashionable to throw around the phrase, "Safe, Sane & Consensual." I have used it many times myself when speaking to the leather public. Yet, as I have done so, there has always been a small corner of my mind that has whispered, very quietly, "Well, yes, but..."

You see, I get past the word "Safe" rather quickly: I don't like hurting others by accident—it seems clumsy and unrefined to me. "Sane" doesn't cause me much of a problem either: I don't suffer from hallucinations, and I am in good contact with reality (fortunately, others around me confirm this).

It is the word "Consensual"—the concept of consent that slows me down. In fact, I happen to know that many players in the SM scene raise an unseen eyebrow when they hear it, but generally, they say nothing.

At endless workshops about SM, the presenters repeatedly stress the need for communication, good negotiation before and during the scene, checking out limits and the like. It is easy to come away from these presentations with the impression that the "correct" whip master, for example, will practically stop after each stroke to see if that one was okay, asking, "Please, Sir Bottom, May I Continue?"

Perhaps, this sort of approach might work for some experimental type scenes, or between novices who are playing together, but I doubt that most guys who are getting "high" with SM work that way together. In short, I suspect that thinking about consent has been too simplistic, and therefore, of limited value.

Many bottoms, especially those who have experience with the more intense end of the stimulation spectrum, report that they need to be pushed past that point which defines their limits. The problem comes up when the Top becomes too responsive to the bottom's arrival at his limit. Many bottoms can't prevent themselves from stopping the scene or slowing it down when they are at (or almost at) their limits—the point where they are no longer able to tolerate a given stimulation, whip strokes, electricity, or whatever. So, bottoms can find themselves stopping a Top before they get where they (the bottoms) want to go. They then come away from the scene saying, "Damn! I wish we had gone just a bit farther even though I know I called a halt to the action—I just couldn't help myself." For a bottom to go this extra distance can sometimes require a Top who will ignore the initial, often involuntary, "stop signs"—up to a point, anyway. (I wonder if this might be the reason that Tops who know how to do this tend to be such desirable play partners among experienced bottoms.)

Perhaps for this reason, some (maybe many, maybe most—I don't know) bottoms have erotic fantasies about themselves that include the element of "being taken" against their will, being used exclusively to pleasure the Dominant/Master/Sadist. Some Tops have the corresponding fantasy which can sound like this in the Top's head: "I want what I want—when I want it—the way I want it. I want it on time, in time, every time with no bullshit. No argument. No resistance. And, I want you to love me for it, but I don't care if you don't."

Although I'm not sure, my suspicion is that this is perhaps what accounts for the prevalence of kidnap and/or rape fantasies among both Tops and bottoms. (Bottoms will generally admit to this fantasy more readily than Tops, by the way.) Non-consensuality is at the core of this fantasy for both Tops and bottoms.

Incidentally, real kidnap, rape, and torture are generally thought to be possible only at the hands of strangers. I have often heard it said that as an SM scenario, these types of scenes won't work if the players are too familiar with each other. I presume that this is because Americans are generally more willing to do violence to strangers than to those with whom we are familiar. (Actual research bears this out, by the way.) In fictional treatments of both rape and kidnap/torture scenes, when the Top is familiar with the victim (bottom now becomes a victim, you will notice), the Top often ends up identifying so strongly with the "plight" of the victim, that the stories can turn into rescues of the hapless bottom.

Additionally, a great many Tops with whom I have discussed these issues report to me that they have a tough time engaging in truly non-consenting, sadistic behaviors with men towards whom they feel a genuine affection. So, I have had "married" Tops say to me, "Take him and go play real hard with him, because I can't and he needs it." It has been my experience that these Tops can't watch their bottoms being heavily played with—it's too hard on Tops emotionally.

Generally, bottoms don't like to shut scenes down. They do it reluctantly! Bottoms will withdraw their consent when the scene stops working and looks like it can't be fixed. This will usually (though not always) happen when they 1) get bored, 2) get too scared, 3) become too exhausted to continue, 4) get angry at the Top for whatever reason, 5) decide their safety has become doubtful, 6) become sick or injured during a scene, or, 7) become neurologically confused by competing stimuli. They can also find themselves involuntarily shutting down scenes when they become over-saturated with some stimulation, even when they are getting "high" on that stimulation. Tops wanting to take the bottom "the whole distance" will need the skills necessary to know when to continue in spite of the stop signals they might be getting from bottom.

It would be nice to just say to Tops, "Leave it to your intuition", but that won't help most Tops because everyone's intuition operates differently, and, regrettably, some Tops simply don't have much to begin with. In the absence of proven and refined intuition, the wisest fall-back tactic is truthful conversation about the bottom's real SM destination. But even with this information, the Top/bottom team is only part way "home."

We can hope that bottoms who have experienced the frustration of stopping scenes before they "arrived" will be able to describe the details of the problem, first for themselves, then later, for cooperative Tops. But bottoms will only have this information if they have bothered to really pay attention to what is happening in their heads when they bail out of the scene prematurely. Bottoms must be willing and able to listen to their own internal feelings and thoughts as they remember what was happening in those scenes they shut down too soon.

My guess is that these bottoms will be unable to get past their tendency to bail out prematurely without this information from inside themselves. Few Tops have the psychological skills necessary to chase down this information by dragging it out of the bottom. It is unreasonable for bottoms to expect Tops to be willing to help with this difficulty until *after* the bottoms have done their own homework on themselves. In fact, it has become my impression that most Tops simply won't play more than once with bottoms who bail out prematurely. Worse, bottoms who bail out too soon can quickly get a reputation among Tops for doing so; the result is predictable.

So, exactly what information can help deal with premature bail outs? Both Top and bottom can be usefully guided by the following data which can only come from inside the bottom:

First, information about what's going on in bottom's head just prior to bailout is a good place to start. Does this bottom say things to himself in his head that scare him out of the scene? Does the progressive loss of control as the scene builds result in a panic that makes bottom grab for control again? Does he tell himself that his physical or emotional safety has become doubtful when it really hasn't? Do thoughts pop into his head that shame his participation in the SM scene? Does he decide the Top is "doing it" wrong? Does he force his concentration away from the scene?

Second, Tops can try to find out exactly how these bottoms have usually gone about shutting down the action prematurely in previous scenes. Do they demand safe words that they end up

194

using when they don't really want to? Do they thrash around in a dangerous manner? Do they start to babble and look like they've lost their minds? Do they scream, "Stop, STOP!", or maybe start swearing at the Top?

Third, wise Tops will ask the bottom's opinion about how they could best cooperate to move past the "sticking point"—the point where bottom says, "No more!", but doesn't really mean it. Possibilities include: 1) slow, gentle persuasion from Top; 2) escalation of the stimulation; 3) a gradual reduction in the stimulation for a short time while bottom catches his breath, so to speak; 4) having his pleas to stop the action simply be ignored; 5) being humiliated for asking that the action stop; 6) "buying" the cessation of the action in say two minutes by agreeing to continue that long with the understanding that it really will end shortly; and many others. Once this information is on the table, the Top/bottom team will have a much better chance of getting where they really want to go with the scene.

Playing in front of others complicates this issue because, in supervised dungeons, Dungeon Masters will intervene in a scene where bottom is calling a halt, but Top is continuing. And there is the added risk that observers will conclude that the continuing Top is an irresponsible player, not to be trusted. Most Tops who play in public are unwilling to risk such a reputation because it can jeopardize their access to bottoms in the future. Tops in such a situation are in a "No-Win" position. They are damned by observers and/or Dungeon Masters if they continue, and damned by their bottom partner if they stop the scene when the bottom calls one of his premature halts to the action. Either circumstance will have the effect of castrating the Top psychologically and possibly number His days in the SM scene.

One solution to this dilemma might be for both Top and bottom to approach the Dungeon Master on duty before the scene begins, and outline together what the Top/bottom team's objective in the scene really is. Dungeon Masters in this situation will need to be warned that bottom's pleas to stop the scene will need to be ignored, at least up to a point. The Dungeon Master could be asked to stand by and directly observe the entire scene as it unfolds. This would put him in a position to signal to observers that the scene in progress was carefully negotiated in advance.

I have also seen bottoms prepare a written sign for all to see that announces something like "Stop Doesn't Mean *STOP*". Observers are then less likely to draw conclusions that might be uncharitable towards the Top. Tops can also consider the inclusion of a gag provided that it does not obstruct breathing.

Another solution I have seen work well in such situations calls for two Tops to play with the bottom in question. Two Tops can support each other through the bottom's attempts to stop the scene prematurely. Still another possibility is to supply the bottom with a supportive companion during the scene. *Sometimes* such a person will have to be in continuous physical contact with the bottom to help him get past the sticking point. Any combination of the above strategies can be used to break through the barrier of the involuntary, premature termination of a scene by the bottom. But unless the players have been completely honest with each other about their objectives for the scene, there is little chance that things will change much or change fast.

Some Straight Talk About Drugs

"No bird soars too high, if he soars with his own wings."

—William Blake, *The Marriage of Heaven and Hell*, 1790-93

It is no accident that all the SM clubs I am familiar with have rules about the use of drugs (including alcohol, of course) at their events. The existence and enforcement of these rules is a tacit acknowledgement that enough members of the SM community not only use drugs but abuse them often enough that policies to handle drug use at SM events have become necessary.

No one likes to mention these facts because we are concerned that an open acknowledgement of drug use in our community will give us a bad name. So, we don't talk openly about drugs much, and the problems continue.

These days, almost any conversation about drugs can quickly turn into a highly charged debate. In this essay, I want to raise some of the issues that surround drug use, in the hope that doing so may help you clarify your own thoughts about them. Drug use is a plenty complicated enough subject to begin with, but coupled with SM, the issues can start to spin out of control fast.

When I use the word "drug" here, I mean any substance that is taken into the body to change the way that we normally think or feel either emotionally or physically. In short, a drug is any substance which changes the way we "read" the world. I *omit* from this definition prescription drugs when used only as directed by a doctor.

Humans, as a group, seem to like to fiddle around with the way the world "reads." It has also been suggested that it may be natural for us to do so based partly on the observation that children all over the world are fond of twirling themselves into a state of temporary dizziness, thus altering their perceptions momentarily.

Even in many so called primitive societies isolated from each other, drugs and drug manufacture have been discovered and woven into the social fabric. From the anthropological data that exist, it does seem clear that it is a human thing to want to alter one's perceptions, one's consciousness in one way or another, but most especially with chemicals, alcohol being the world-wide favorite.

So, it then becomes all the more necessary to distinguish between drug use and drug abuse. One handy way to approach this very important distinction is to think in terms of side effects. All drugs have side effects. Let me explain: When you get a headache, your perception of the world changes, and you become uncomfortable. If you decide to fix the discomfort by taking the drug, aspirin, you unconsciously make a decision to accept the risks of the possible side effects in order to receive the benefit.

In the case of aspirin, you "decide" to risk minor bleeding in your stomach, ringing in your ears, a change in ability of your blood to clot normally, and other side effects. Aspirin, for most people, is a low risk drug because the benefit comes at doses low enough to avoid the unpleasant side effects. So, with aspirin, we like the relationship between what it costs us to take the drug compared to the benefit we get from taking the drug.

Now let's move this discussion into a leather bar, and order a drink. Most of us drink without thinking much about it. We go to a bar because we want something—maybe several things. For the most part, we go there because we think it will feel better to be there than any other place for various reasons. One of the first things that happens when we go into the bar is that we decide whether to stay, or turn around and walk out. This happens fast, and the decision is influenced by too many factors to list here. But, the second decision we make is usually what to order from the bartender.

Bars sell lots of stuff, and we know this. This is the instant that we decide whether to change the chemistry of our perception processes or not. It is in this split second that we weigh the costs of the drug against the benefit of the drug. The cost/benefit relationship with alcohol is pretty good for the first or second drink for most people. Beyond that, the cost associated with side effects starts to rise rapidly, and can quickly overtake the benefit payoff. Indeed, with more and more drinks, the benefit payoff starts to actually drop off rapidly just as the cost part goes way up.

Because we are all greedy, we want all benefit and no cost. But it doesn't work that way with alcohol, or any other drug for that matter. We use drugs to solve problems, and very small problems often get solved with very small amounts of drugs. But, at the same time, we must be sensitive to the moment when the drug solution turns into the drug problem.

For example, we go out for a good time, and end up in the drunk tank, with a drunk driving charge. Or, we go to a fisting party thinking we might take just a little crystal to help us through the night, and we end up wrung out and depressed three or four days later having lost eight pounds, and somehow we know the same thing will happen next weekend.

Not being able to figure out the cost/benefit relationship or not being able to act on this information in a self protective way, is what distinguishes drug use from drug abuse.

Most folks are very clear about what the "benefit" of their favorite drug(s) might be. Drug abusers are poor at learning what the real costs are, partly because some costs are hidden, and abusers don't really want to know the truth about what their drug intake costs them. Once abusers become actually addicted to a drug (including alcohol, of course) they are indifferent to the costs, obsessed with only the benefits.

People are not usually very clear about the cost part of the picture. Let me take a moment to list what I think are the most important of the overlooked costs:

First and foremost is the fact that when people take drugs of all kinds, especially alcohol, their ability to assess risks is diminished. It is harder to pay attention to, and to enforce, safer

199

sex guidelines after four drinks than after two. Nowadays, getting loaded may lower your guard in sexual encounters to the point where you might allow yourself to bend your own rules, such that you become exposed to HIV, or willing to tolerate incompetent SM technique.

We used to think that a "problem drinker" was someone who got sloshed regularly. Now we know that a "problem drinker" may simply be someone who isn't comfortable in a social situation without first consuming a quantity of alcohol that will also make him indifferent to how he gets fucked. For these guys, four drinks can be life threatening—make no mistake about it!

Second, there is little dispute now among medical professionals that all recreational drugs and some medical drugs are hard on the immune system to one degree or another. Amphetamines, which includes cocaine/crack, crystal/speed, Praeludin and others, are probably the most hostile to one's immune system. If you are HIV positive, the danger from these drugs is very much increased. Also, these drugs are hell on your liver and kidneys.

Recreational drugs always change the way that we register body stress, including pain. Bottoms will often tell me that they take drugs to increase their SM tolerance. They believe that it is important for them to have high pain tolerances to be attractive to experienced Tops. Unfortunately, some bottoms seem to confuse being a *good* bottom with being a *heavy* bottom. There is a big difference!

Most Tops I discuss this with have told me that a bottom on drugs is a lot more work to play with than one who is not. It takes more effort to reach their limits, and most Tops aren't that eager to work that hard for anyone more than once.

Tops also complain that they don't get "true" reactions from a bottom on drugs. It's as though they have to reach for the bottom through the drug influence. Typically, a Top in a scene needs to get accurate information from a bottom's body in order to skillfully lead the scene in the directions that will reveal the bottom's true capacities and tastes. Drugs make the discovery process cloudy and imprecise.

Also, Tops who are into control stuff report that when a bottom has taken some drug(s), it can feel to the Tops like the bottom has placed himself somehow beyond the reach of the Top. They can feel like they are at the mercy of the drug that is acting on the bottom they are trying to play with.

I do not mean to suggest that bottoms are the ones taking all the drugs. Tops take them too, occasionally with disastrous results. I mentioned earlier that drugs cloud one's ability to accurately assess risk. A Top on a drug may be more inclined to try something for the first time, pretend that he knows what he is doing, and get in over his head. Tops on drugs also are at risk for compromising their own safer sex standards, and becoming exposed to dangerous diseases.

Since I work primarily with guys in the scene, one of the things that has come to disturb me more and more is the extent to which men have come to associate sex with drug taking. By now, I have met many who just cannot play without taking some drug or other. When they decide to stop taking drugs, they find that they can't make sex work, so sex seems to go out the window at the same time. Then, the time bomb starts ticking for sure!

When I have taken drug histories, what often turns up is that guys started out by using small amounts of drugs to achieve enhancement of the sexual experience. When we like something, we tend to repeat it, so using drugs as a sexual enhancement becomes a pattern, a habit, if you will. After a while, guys get to the point where they routinely include drugs as an integral part of the sexual event.

Most people discover that they can get away with taking a small amount of whatever, enjoy themselves, and not become raving addicts overnight. Then they become curious about other drugs and/or the effect of somewhat larger doses. The process of drug experimentation has begun. Typically, this process continues until the person has a bad experience he feels was caused by the drug, or begins to suspect that he is overdoing it. The suspicion may come in various ways. There may be legal troubles, including arrest. He might notice that the financial outlay has become significant, and that there is now a "drug budget." A potential play partner may reject him when he is unwilling to play without the drug.

Friends may sound the alarm. Maybe he is missing too much work on Mondays, and maybe sometimes Tuesdays as well. His health may deteriorate. He gets uptight when he can't seem to make a drug buy—not usually a problem with alcohol since it's always available in most places.

The moments of suspicion are usually the first time a drug user must begin to consciously examine the cost/benefit relationship of drug taking to see if he has become an abuser. If he is worried enough about himself, he may try to pull back from, or discontinue his drug taking, and he may be successful all by himself. If he keeps slipping back into his old, worrisome using patterns, he may think about getting involved with a recovery program or consult a therapist for help. If he does neither, his life is probably in danger, and perhaps the lives of others as well.

We on the sexual frontier spend a lot of time telling outsiders and each other that we must all protect everybody's right to be who they want to be. We talk about the American freedom to explore our diversity, and we use this reasoning to fight the repression of our lifestyle by religious and political conservatives, by other gay people, and by closeted kinky people as well. This theme of self-determination is central to this discussion of drugs. "It's my life," we say, "and I can do whatever I choose to do with it, and it's none of your business." Caution is in order here, because the right to experiment with drugs is also the right to destroy one's self.

When I am going into a scene with someone, I have a right to know what he has taken, because his right to take a drug ends at the point where my safety, sanity and consent may be at risk.

The Mental Side Of Playing "Safe" & "Sane"

These days, it is very stylish to throw the words, safe, sane, consensual around when we are talking about the SM/leather/fetish sex style. As a "community" it has been fairly easy for us to take up the matter of what constitutes safety from a physiological point of view and, consequently, there have been a host of articles, workshops and demonstrations that convey good information about how to avoid accidental or unwanted physical injury in a scene.

Most players in the scene who have taken the time and energy to educate themselves now feel fairly secure with the safety of their technique. But when we move on to the issues of achieving a scene that is "safe and sane" from a mental or emotional viewpoint, the sense of security can vanish in a heartbeat. To begin with, the definition of "sanity" is sometimes slippery and hard to pin down. Mental health care providers either retreat to the position of "I know it when I see it," or rely on the current manual of mental disorders with all its carefully constructed definitions of mental ailments.

For kinky people, this presents special difficulties because the currently accepted manual of mental disorders (DSM IIIR) classes all of our favorite (kinky) erotic pastimes under the general heading of "Sexual Disorders." One of the tests for the diagnosis of "Sexual Disorder" includes the statement, "The person has acted on these urges [take your pick], or is markedly distressed by them." So, for mainstream mental health care providers, we all suffer from a "Sexual Disorder" if we have acted on these urges.

Remember, homosexuality was also considered a "Sexual Disorder," and it was not until 1973 with a ruling from the American Psychiatric Association, that the professional view of homosexuality changed. Overnight, many millions of people were suddenly no longer officially "ill." It was better than a good day at Lourdes.

My point here is that the definition of what constitutes mental health (or illness) is something that emerges from the socio-cultural and historical context in which that definition is made. In Salem, Massachusetts once upon a time, the consensus was that those whose behavior did not conform were witches. Those afflicted with witching were either dunked in water or burned to drive out the possessing spirits, and no one thought this practice strange. Among the Sambia, a New Guinea tribe of "primitives," a man is considered abnormal unless he offers his penis to a prepubescent boy for sucking. This tribe believes that, without this gift, the boys cannot grow into full manhood. In this context, a male adult would be considered disordered, deviant if he refused to have his cock sucked by a boy!

My guess is that in time, as mental health care professionals become more educated about kinky behaviors, their view of us will become more refined, and their definitions will begin to distinguish those of us who engage in these behaviors in healthy ways from those who do not. But for now, we cannot rely on the mental health profession for guidance in the matter of what constitutes mentally healthy ways to be kinky because they are still far too ignorant about us and our behaviors to be of use to us.

As a person who, as of this writing, has spent upwards of 45,000 hours in the therapy room treating practicing sadomasochists, I have developed a number of guidelines, viewpoints and biases, if you will, with regard to the issues of emotional and psychological safety and "sanity" among sadomasochists. It has become my view that there can be real risks to mental health and emotional stability when individuals approach their SM encounters in the belief that they are an appropriate setting in which to accomplish the resolution of anger issues, guilt issues, and/or suppressed or repressed issues concerning child abuse (physical, emotional or sexual).

I also become suspicious about the psychological motives

for one's participation in the SM scene when I begin hearing reports from clients about the onset of strong depressions immediately following all or most of their SM scenes or fantasies about scenes. I am similarly concerned when I begin hearing about unwanted injuries (including marks), reports about a "helpless" attraction to another person, flashback memories from traumatic childhood days, the need always to use drugs or alcohol before or during a scene, the inability of individuals to form healthy romantic relationships in spite of their wish to do so, the wish to be or have a partner who is totally dependant on their partner, and others.

A second set of issues that concern me in the therapy room arises when I begin to suspect "hidden agendas" as the motivation for participation in the SM scene. Some of these might be: the wish of an otherwise non-kinky person to please a kinky lover, the wish to die in a scene when it comes from a physically healthy person, or the wish to be taken against one's will. Other agendas of concern might be the need to establish a reputation in the leather "community," the need to find a social niche, the need to hurt a former partner through a new connection with someone kinky, the need to connect with the Devil or an extraterrestrial, to follow orders broadcast into one's head from elsewhere, to fulfill a prophesy or prediction made by a parent/friend/lover, or because the one we are playing with reminds us of someone else.

When such as these are the themes of participation in the SM scene, the SM is usually not the objective itself. It is, instead, placed in the service of some other purpose. I fear that when this happens, the SM is being used as a tool, corrupted if you will, to accomplish something else which may not be psychologically beneficial, and may even be harmful.

A third area of concern has to do with the development of an hypnotic state during a scene which can envelope one or both players. When hypnotic states occur during the SM encounter, there is a risk that material from the unconscious portion of the mind may flood into the conscious, aware part of the mind, overwhelming one or both players with unwanted recollections from the past.

Most players lack the experience necessary to handle an emotional crisis of this kind in the playroom, often completely without warning. Occasionally, such events result in serious psychological trauma. Most experienced players, many intermediate players and a few novice players know this sort of thing can sometimes happen. They understand that the SM encounter can be used as a mechanism to alter one's consciousness (which we like most of the time).

During such altered states of consciousness—when hypnotic states can occur—both the conscious and unconscious mind can be left in a less well-defended state than usual. It is at these times that players may find that they are much more vulnerable than they had ever intended to be. This is not necessarily a bad thing, because part of the scene is playing with vulnerability. But at these times, there is sometimes a risk that ideas and attitudes can be introduced into the mind that may not have been there before. This sort of thing can violate consent before you know it. In bottoms, already low self-esteem can be reinforced if verbally abusive language is hurled into an unguarded mind. Tops in such a state can get to feeling like they can do nothing wrong.

A good general rule of thumb is that an SM experience that leaves you feeling emotionally refreshed is one that you need not have concerns about. The ones that leave you in emotional turmoil, or leave you with unwanted psychological pain are the ones to pay closer attention to.

Following are some guidelines that can serve to protect your mental health and emotional safety in connection with the SM scene:

1) Don't lie to yourself about what you want in a scene, or why you play. Most people who get into emotional trouble in scenes do so because they don't know themselves very well.

2) If you don't feel good emotionally after a scene, try to find out the reason by spending some honest time with yourself, writing about it if necessary. It will help to get very clear with yourself about what you liked in the scene, and what you

didn't. This is not an opportunity for Top bashing. As a bottom, you share responsibility for what happens in a scene.

3) If you know that you have specific areas of emotional vulnerability that you don't want to play with, you can discuss these with your partner before the scene just as you would discuss physical problems.

4) If you have a sense, even a vague feeling that someone might not be emotionally safe to play with, then don't until you learn more about him, and maybe more about your own attractions to him.

5) If a scene is going in an emotional direction that you feel uneasy about or in danger from, either steer the scene in another direction, or bail out as delicately as you can.

6) Be very cautious about your use of drugs and alcohol when playing. Be watchful to see if you find yourself falling into a pattern of substance use regularly, prior to or during play. Consider it a serious warning if you regularly have trouble remembering what happened in the scene.

7) Pay attention to what you hear about others who develop a reputation for playing in emotionally dangerous ways. But also remember that there is malicious gossip about people, which may not be true. Just check it out for yourself.

8) If you become suspicious about your emotional process regarding your involvement in the SM scene, first do some honest writing to yourself about your concerns. If you still have questions after doing this, talk to a trusted friend. Then seek some appropriate professional assistance, if you are still doubtful.

9) Don't hesitate to get to know the people you want to play with so that you can check out their own emotional stability.

10) Don't take your wounded inner child into the playroom except maybe for strictly sensual or playful sorts of scenes. SM is for consenting adults and is no place for children, especially an injured one that may be inside you. If you like to play with pain trips or heavy verbal abuse trips, leave your kid at the door when you walk in.

Humiliation:
What's In It For You?

Just as there are healthy and unhealthy ways to fly airplanes and ride motorcycles, likewise, there are healthy and unhealthy ways to be into SM. Doing planes, bikes and kink in unhealthy ways can get you dead or injured—fast or slow, depending. Naturally, this raises the issue of what exactly is healthy SM.

Any activity which adds something to who we are—enhances us—I call healthy. Admittedly, this is, and must remain a subjective assessment. As a psychotherapist working with kinky men, I have observed that those who do SM such that they feel (subjectively) enhanced are happier than those who are self-destructive, guilty, angry, depressed or scared by what they do in their erotic lives.

Since anything powerful (love, fire, nuclear energy, politics, medicine, SM) can create as well as destroy, it is, I believe, useful to examine our involvement in SM to see that it remains a creative element in our lives. My bias in this article is that I support what is creative in a person's life, and oppose what proves to be destructive. We must each define these words for ourselves.

Personal ads that I see soliciting scenes or relationships of one kind or another occasionally mention the word "humiliation." Bottoms say they crave it, or Tops require that bottoms be "into" it as a condition of responding to an ad. Other ads code this interest by using the initials V/A (standing for verbal abuse, but when I first read it, I thought it meant vacuum action). I have decided that it's time for me to share my observations concerning humiliation as a relationship dynamic.

First, it is important to distinguish what happens in a single encounter from what goes on in a scene occurring in the context

209

of some kind of ongoing relationship. A relationship is taken here to mean two or more persons having an ongoing emotional and SM involvement with some sort of negotiated commitment.

In many ways, there is less at stake in a scene between strangers than between, say, lovers or a Master and slave. If a scene between strangers doesn't work, or collapses for some reason, well, it's just another scene that failed. But, have a scene fail between players who are in a relationship, and the fallout can last for months in some cases.

What has all this to do with humiliation? Well, getting humiliated by a stranger seems to have a very different flavor than getting humiliated by someone you care for, who is important to you. The words of a stranger may not slice as deeply. They can be enjoyed for their erotic impact tonight and (probably) be forgotten tomorrow.

A partner's humiliations, in contrast, can be honed to sharpness by intimate knowledge—lasting wounds sometimes result. A stranger is less likely to know where real wounds could be opened, so serious injuries to Self are less likely.

I bring all this up because in relationships, a deeply and regularly humiliated bottom can quickly become a very depressed bottom. "You-are-not-OK" type messages can take root in the fertile soil deep within the Self. This is especially true in young bottoms, or those who may be on shaky psychological footing to begin with. And, guess what? Depressed bottoms usually aren't much fun to be with! At least, not for long.

I do not mean to suggest that humiliation in relationships always produces depressed bottoms, but I see it so often in my practice that I have concluded that there is a real risk. There is a real difference between hot talk and serious humiliation.

Tops who insist on real humiliation, and want relationships, come into treatment complaining about their inability to find and keep "good" bottoms. A closer examination often reveals that they are looking for a psychologically indestructible bottom who will take them and their humiliations seriously.

Tops sometime report that they long for someone to "break"

as part of their fantasy. I have found that when "you-are-not-OK" messages are part of the "breaking" process, the bottom's spirit also breaks, and depression is a frequent result. The Tops who break bottoms without "you-are-not-OK" messages have learned how to end up with proud and devoted partners, spirit intact.

What is also true, however, is that some bottoms like the feelings of humiliation as part of the sexual experience. How can these needs be met in an ongoing relationship without courting the problems of depression? Some partners have solved this dilemma in very creative ways. For example, bottom only gets into heavy-duty humiliation trips *outside* the relationship. Or, more interestingly, Tops do or say things they (Tops) consider humiliating but which bottoms don't read as humiliation.

For example, Top may make bottom wear a collar in public because Top considers that doing so (considering public reaction) *is* humiliation, no matter what the bottom thinks. Bottom, on the other hand, may feel proud to wear his Top's collar.

Another example: Some men would be unspeakably humiliated if they were made to wear a dress, while others would adore to do it (depending on the dress, of course!). No such solutions could be worked out (it could be stumbled upon, though) without careful communication between the partners as to what this stuff really feels like.

There are Tops who *must* deliver their humiliations to bottoms who *do* experience deep and genuine humiliation. I have found that these men do get involved in relationships, but usually they are with strictly vanilla partners. The Tops don't want any lover who would consistently tolerate such abuse, and the bottoms don't want to be crushed consistently, so they choose non-kinky partners.

My pet theory about all this is that humiliation as an erotic theme often impedes, if not prevents, male-to-male bonding, and may even be used as defense against the intimacy that relationships usually imply. Other sorts of common SM erotic themes, by contrast, seem to enhance such bonding.

For example, a Top who sees himself as Protector and Benevolent Despot usually wants to play with the finest manimals* he can find, and perhaps even improve them through his superior stewardship. One feels the possibilities for bonding here more than in the "you no-good faggot-queer" style of erotic interplay.

I worry about the Top who consistently likes to play with "piece-of-shit" bottoms. I wonder how he feels about himself (really) if inferiors are all he lets himself play with. What does a bottom do in his head in order to fall in love with such a person? Agree to be shit?

Clearly, including humiliation as an erotic theme between partners produces a loaded situation, and can have potentially fateful consequences for relationships. My advice for partners who want to—or must—play with this sort of fire is this: Talk together as honestly as possible about fantasy versus actual emotional reality, then proceed cautiously. Get feedback from each other at each step of the way. Stay real and respect limits!

* Thank you Jack Fritcher.

Punishment:
Proceed With Caution!

My object all sublime
I shall achieve in time
To let the punishment fit the crime
The punishment fit the crime.

—W.S. Gilbert, *The Mikado, II*

We come into the SM scene by many routes. Some arrive by way of bondage, others through dominance and submission, still others through their child abuse experiences. For others, however, the association of "pain" with pleasure first occurred during or just following punishment(s) for misdeeds committed during childhood, adolescence, or, more rarely, in adulthood. A great many men have also reported being aroused while watching punishment scenes in movies, or reading about them in literature.

For these and other reasons, punishment themes will sometimes take a prominent position in people's SM sexuality. When these themes express themselves in relationships, however, all hell can sometimes break loose, because psychologically dangerous forces often come into play. I want to warn you about them now.

First, let's get clear as to which behaviors I am talking about. In the "bad boy" style, a masochistic bottom makes a mistake or bungles something, and gets punished by a Top in some way that is physically painful or humiliating, and maybe even erotic. If the "mistake" is trivial, or the punishment blatantly unfair (according to the bottom), there can be lots of emotional pain and stress as well.

The Top counterpart is the guy who is always on the

213

lookout for the error in a bottom's ways. If the Top doesn't find enough mistakes to justify a scene, he can make them up, or set the bottom up so that mistakes are inevitable. Usually, this is all done under the guise of "training" or "discipline."

Think about this for a minute, and you can begin to see the problems. First of all, in the bottom's head, he only gets what he desires (to be played with) when he fails. This rewards his ineptness, and does not reinforce skill and capability. Additionally, charges of ineptitude cause people to feel bad about themselves, whereas feeling capable and competent makes people feel good about themselves.

Followed to its logical conclusion, after a while, a Top would end up with a bottom who couldn't do anything right, ever! In fact, this sometimes happens. Other bottoms learn only to fuck up when they are horny. This then provokes (manipulates) the Top and a scene starts—maybe. The bottom then gets to play, but pays the price of believing that he has done something "bad," or is, himself, "bad." He must *believe* he has done something bad in order to take the Top and his punishment seriously.

In this way, many bottoms have come to lose their self respect and self esteem in exchange for sexual fulfillment. Critical, punishing Tops have made them believe that they can do nothing right, and that they are total fuck-ups. This view of themselves is systematically reinforced with sex and orgasm—pretty powerful reinforcement, I'd say. To make matters worse, these bottoms can begin to get very depressed, and therefore not much fun to be around, even for the Tops who create them.

Interestingly, many of the "punish" Tops that I have worked with clinically have explained that it is all for the good of the bottom. Each one claims he is teaching something important about life that the bottom has somehow missed earlier. None makes any comments, initially, about his hard dick, as though that were unimportant to the explanation of his wish to punish.

Just for you psychology buffs, here are some ideas about what is often going on inside, which allows all this to happen in the first place. For the bottom, punishment may recreate the situation in which he may have come to associate pain and pleasure in childhood. Suddenly, the whipping (or whatever) is justified and "makes sense" because he has been "bad." It feels bad emotionally and good physically, but he *does* like the attention—very confusing to the mind.

In the Top's own head, he may be recreating an identification with an admired, punishing or strict relative, or an identification with an admired character in a movie or book—the Sheriff of Nottingham, for example, or Captain Nemo. Top understands that, when he can find errors, he can do something that will make his dick hard—an idea with appeal. Psychologically, the most common reason that he goes through all this is to explain and justify his sadism to himself. "Well, after all," the Top says, "he fucked up again, and I just *had* to do something."

Numerous hours in the therapy room with "bad boy" bottoms and "punish" Tops has led me to some interesting discoveries. For the most part, it seems that these guys can't permit themselves to let their needs for hurting or being hurt come out, without *first* establishing a pretext which would be acceptable to society in general. Otherwise, they might feel guilty for enjoying themselves in such an unconventional way. The punishment set up provides both of them with the excuse they need to get down to it. So, unconsciously, we get, "I can hit him when he is bad," and "he can hit me when he thinks I have been bad." It's all OK then. There is nothing twisted or sick.

I suspect that these men go through these mental gymnastics because we are socialized to believe that it is only OK to "hurt" someone else when they have broken the law or committed a sin. We are also socialized to believe that it is only OK for someone else to "hurt" us when we have done a bad thing.

Sadly, for a smaller number of others, it is all just thinly disguised child abuse done with an overgrown child. Both Top and bottom suffer those associated ills when this is the situation.

It is truly hard for me to imagine a healthy relationship in which a Top is constantly scrutinizing his partner's behavior for punishable mistakes, and a bottom who has (or thinks he has) figured out how to get played with by making mistakes. Or, if the bottom is not horny, or does not want to play, he must then go to the emotional trouble of trying extra hard *not* to fuck something up, and bring down an unwanted scene on himself. (This is fun? This feels good? This is quality time?)

One reason I doubt the health of such an arrangement is that the "bad boy" bottom can't come to see himself as a competent, effective man in the world, and still get his sexual needs met. I have stated my chief bias about SM sexuality in an earlier article: I support those behaviors that add to who we are and make us feel better about ourselves, and oppose behaviors that do the opposite.

Put differently, research shows us that something called "cognitive dissonance" creates unhealthy psychologies. Simply speaking, this term describes a state of dangerous internal mental conflict, which occurs when the mind tries to hold contradictory emotional information. It is clear to me that the punishment scene can create cognitive dissonance in a number of ways. For example, the rest of the world gives us rewards when we do a good job. If we have to make an exception in our sexuality, that creates dissonance and the trouble that goes with it. Another source of dissonance in the punishment game is that Tops do (occasionally) make mistakes of all kinds. More dissonance happens in both their heads when Top does not get punished for his mistakes. He is confronted with his double standards, while the bottom must try somehow to look the other way. In this situation, couples report that their relationships take on an increasingly unreal quality, making it difficult to sustain the connected feelings that are essential to the maintenance of SM relationships.

Of course, everyone makes mistakes because we are all human, and no one is perfect. Mistakes are a natural part of living, and an opportunity for growth, self awareness and development. They need to be seen in a positive light because they afford us the opportunity to learn important things about the world. To hand out physical punishment or verbal abuse when "mistakes" are made is not supportive or educational except perhaps in the most primitive way.

Endless studies reveal that corporal punishment does not work to modify behavior as well as other more supportive methods. This means that the behavior modification excuse used to justify physical punishment for misdeeds, by calling it SM, just doesn't wash.

Lots of men get into the punishment scene because they cannot allow themselves to do this stuff simply because it feels so damn good all by itself. In their value system, pure pleasure is not considered sufficient justification to engage in what vanilla folks (both straight and gay) would call "hurting" behaviors. Sadomasochists call it fun, and it is for us—when we do it right.

Most kinky guys don't feel the need to create a socially acceptable pretext for doing anything in their sexuality. They have freed themselves from vanilla values so completely that what society would say is just not important anymore. They play just because it feels good.

My view of the punishment scene today is that it is the way that some SM people manage (but don't resolve) an internal conflict between their sexual impulses and social rules. The emotional fallout is so great though, that I am not at all clear that it is worth it for them to pander to the internal vanilla values that tug at them.

Lastly, there is a punishment style that does not cause any of the troubles mentioned above, and it is remarkably useful in correcting unwanted behaviors. That punishment consists of varying degrees of abandonment/withdrawal—a bottom's worst fear, in my opinion. Ignoring a bottom is a much clearer signal than a slap when a Top is unhappy. The slap is a mixed message—anything that is physical is a mixed message. To slap for punishment one moment and slap as a reward, or as an "I love you" message the next is so-o-o confusing to the psychology of a masochistic bottom.

Reserving SM behaviors for horny times and feel-good

situations sends a consistent message to bottoms, and does not confuse them. If they are good, play with them and have a good time. If they are displeasing, tell them why and how, and send them away for a while, or go elsewhere and play with someone pleasing.

I feel strongly that anyone in the scene who is committed to the principles of Safe, Sane, Consensual is in danger of violating the "Sane" part when he uses or invites physical punishment to correct unwanted behavior. Doing so constitutes a real threat to the self esteem and confidence of many bottoms, and thus places their mental health at risk. I can't support any scene that risks any kind of health, can you?

Part Four

CATAPULTING TOWARD TRANSFORMATION

Editor's Note On
Catapulting Toward Transformation

There was no Part Four intended for this book. It came about organically, growing against the plans I shared with Baldwin and his publisher. This section is composed of an essay on the direction from ordinary experience, through SM, to ecstasy; one on the dark, nearly-secret stirrings in the depths of SM Tops; and a fragment from a third which returns us to the all-embracing attitude expressed in the book's opening essay, "A Second Coming Out." These pieces refused, for reasons that may be obvious, to be forced into close companionship with the ones in any other section of the book. They also refused to be separated from one another.

It seemed for a day or so that what I considered a very significant group of essays were going to have to be distributed in half-acceptable slots throughout the manuscript. Then things got worse. It became clear that most of the final essay appeared as a subsection of "A Second Coming Out." Panic drove me to call the author with a plea for help with what I called "an editor's nightmare." Emergency surgery was performed on one essay. Then, within half an hour, Baldwin and I watched my "problem children" mature, and give birth to Part Four. Baldwin looked at the new product and, by the magic of naming it, made it meaningful.

Here human relationships, our leather communities, and SM experience are taken as givens. The subject, then, becomes a sort of "what for and what next." For Baldwin, as you will see, these are descriptives, not questions.

To Ecstasy And Beyond: One Road Map

Talk honestly with bottoms about what spoils a scene for them, and you will discover that this can sometimes happen when Tops become predictable, don't push limits, are too easy-going, easily manipulated, and the like. A number of bottoms to whom I listen also tell me that unless they feel a bit nervous during a scene, it is unlikely to work well for them. Some have said that the nervousness must get close to fear for the scene to work, and a few tell me outright that they need to be scared shitless before they can get "high" in the scene.

When I press for more information about this, I almost always learn that these bottoms do not want to be nervous or scared about the safety aspects of the Top's technique or his sanity. For example, they don't want to worry that a dildo might be contaminated or that a suspension device is doubtful, or that the Top is going to go crazy and lose control of himself. These things don't lead to the "fun" kind of nervous for most bottoms.

For these bottoms, "fun" starts to happen when they are forced to confront their own "limits." What *exactly* does that mean? Once they can stop worrying about *safe & sane*, bottoms are then able to concentrate on the stimulation they are receiving—whip strokes, hot wax, feathers, or whatever. Many bottoms seem to need the anxiety that happens as they approach and arrive face to face with their own capacity to deal with stimulation. As the stimulation levels increase, bottoms wrestle with the assimilation process as they struggle to digest that stimulation. It becomes a war between two parts of the bottom: one part wants to put a stop to the pushy stimulation, and the other wants to master it and get beyond it. "Can I take it, or will it break me?"

223

When bottoms are able (allowed) to assimilate and recover from each stimulation *at their own pace*, then the scene hums along. Bottom's endorphins start to flood his brain chemistry, and his stimulation limits generally increase as this happens. He gets "high" on the stimulation itself.

But when Top stimulates faster and/or more intensely than the bottom can assimilate, bottom's body and head start moving toward overload—toward what I call the threshold of tolerability. A bottom can be moved to this threshold instantly, say with a single, very intense whip stroke, a needle in the wrong spot, or a quantity of hot wax delivered all at once.

Or, a bottom can be moved to this threshold very slowly, gradually increasing the intensity of the stimulations. Tops can do this thing depending on which whip they use next, and how, and where they use it. Or by dripping wax strategically and at a certain rate, or whatever.

Experience has shown me that bottoms who are moved along toward their threshold of tolerability more slowly will ultimately be able to tolerate more stimulation of higher intensity than those who are moved there quickly. This is generally even more true for bottoms with less practice at assimilating and recovering from physical stimulations. Conversely, a few very experienced bottoms have developed the skill necessary to get well connected to heavier stimulation almost right from the start, but they are much more rare.

Put simply, in terms of intensity, if you want to go farther and stay there longer, as a Top, you will generally need to go slower to give bottom time to assimilate and recover, or else risk that the bottom will bail out of the scene—withdraw consent. If you want to learn to go farther as a bottom, you will generally need to choose Tops who are greedy, but not speedy; who know how to hold their greed in check long enough for you (bottom) to find your way into your sweet spot—the place where the stimulation generates the endorphin flood. Once Top and bottom have arrived in sync at the bottom's sweet spot, they can really start to play with the uppermost limits of the bottom's threshold of tolerability, and maybe even begin to make excursions into the land of Ecstasy.

Ecstasy? Where is that and how do I know I'm there when I'm there? As bottom reaches his threshold of tolerability, his body usually becomes more and more involuntary; twitching, shaking, struggling, spitting, whimpering, laughing, yelling, screaming, giggling, even pissing and shitting or vomiting are all possible reactions. At or just past the threshold of tolerability, bottom simply loses control of himself (his Self), his muscles, and his voice; he becomes pure reaction. This place past the threshold of tolerability is known as Ecstasy. There are two ways to get there in the SM scene: one is through pain, and the other through pleasure.

For this discussion, I will call the Ecstasy of pain, Agony, and I will call the Ecstasy of pleasure, ...well, we don't really have a word in English for it. Maybe, "Delight," but that doesn't really get it either—too soft. Whether you journey to Ecstasy via the high road of pleasure or the low road of pain, you end up in a place called Joy if the trip is successful.

The folks for whom the letters S & M stand for *sensuality* and *mutuality* will generally stick to the pleasure road in their scenes, engaging in bondage, fisting, sensual whipping, wax play, or abrasion scenes. The folks for whom the letters S & M stand for *sadism* and *masochism* will tend to prefer scenes where the intensity of the stimulations can be stronger, perhaps bull whips, the heavier electrical toys, needle scenes, fire and/or ice, to name a few.

In my experience, most of us start our scenes down the pleasure road and stay there until one of the players, either the Top or the bottom, invites the other to begin to shift onto the pain road. For the bottom, this invitation is usually given with cues to the Top in the form of begging, body language, or sounds. For the Top, this invitation is usually given by turning up the intensity of the stimulation and supporting the bottom through the assimilation and recovery process. If the increased stimulation didn't work for the bottom, he will try to return the scene to more comfortable ground, which may or may not work for the Top.

225

The vast majority of scenes that I have been in or witnessed start down the pleasure road, and then slowly shift to the pain road until either the bottom saturates in Agony or the Top becomes tired or bored. At that point, the scene will either shift back to the pleasure road for a while or it will end in either a slow cooling down period or crash with a bang. If it cools down, it may be over for good, or it may start up again after a rest.

Most bottoms can tolerate Agony (the pain road) only for very short periods of time (milli-seconds) if at all. Agony is a scary place where one loses his sense of self altogether. My guess is that most bottoms fantasize about the experience of losing themselves in pain, but they want to approach it all very carefully. They want Tops who can provide this experience under controlled circumstances. Bottom wants Top to *take* the (self) control that he (the bottom) must surrender as he reaches and/or crosses the threshold into Agony.

In a scene where the stimulation is primarily physical rather than mental, this almost always means secure bondage just for starters. Bottoms thrashing around in Agony are dangerous to themselves and anyone else who happens to be near. Bottoms in Agony can't hear or respond to commands until the Agony passes. In fact, most become blind—literally cannot see even though their eyes might be open. Agony obliterates the ability to process information that arrives at the brain from the senses, except for what comes from pain receptors.

Bottoms who develop a taste for agony *and* have learned to surrender to the bliss of it can have a reaction that looks very different from the thrashing kind. They often become quite still, or move only very slowly, as if in a dream/trance, or as though they are floating. They can float this way until the stimulation changes in some dramatic way, until the stimulation stops and they recover, or until they become exhausted and collapse.

My experience suggests that bottoms are much more likely to find their way into the bliss of Agony when the Top has taken them there slowly and gradually. If they are floating in their Agony and the stimulation is altered dramatically, say for example, a bull whip scene is suddenly switched to an electrical scene, the floating bottom will usually crash out of his trance-like state and probably become confused and/or angry. This is because the central nervous system adjusts to one kind of stimulation and sustains the endorphin pump on that kind of stimulation. If the method of stimulation is changed, the pump stops abruptly as the nervous system is startled by the new input.

Though most of them don't know it, this is the reason that Tops tend to only offer the bottom's central nervous system one and only one kind of stimulation at a time. Skilled Tops have learned the hard way that it is next to impossible to get a bottom "high" on endorphins by throwing two or more kinds of stimulation at his brain chemistry *simultaneously,* say, for example, heavy tit clamps and bullwhips together, or needles and very hot wax. When differing types of strong stimulation compete for the bottom's attention, an annoying confusion in the brain chemistry is the usual result.

Most bottoms, especially those with some experience, will know when their endorphin pump is a pumpin'. When they notice it, they are likely to give some cues to the Top that "they have arrived." Partly, they do this to let the Top know that he has succeeded, that he has found the keys to the kingdom. But they also do this in the hopes that by encouraging the Top, he will not do anything to change the method or manner of stimulation! The endorphin pump is elusive prey for both Top and bottom. Bottoms know the mental and physical environment the Top has created—which generated the endorphin pump—is a delicate one, and easily disturbed. So bottoms will sometimes go to great lengths to prevent it's disturbance.

This is what accounts for comments like, "Can the music be softer?" "May I move my arm?" "Sir, the light is shining in my eyes and it's hard to see you." "The right restraint isn't as tight as the left one." These sorts of remarks are made in the hopes that the bottom can adjust and perfect the environment of the endorphin pump, so that the scene can go to a "higher level" without distractions which might compete with the Top's stimulations for bottom's attention.

Essentially, my reason for spelling all this out is that I am greedy. I usually want to squeeze out everything that a bottom has in him. I have come to believe that I get much more out of bottoms, and the scenes I have with them, when I keep all these things in mind. Actually, I don't really keep these issues in the forefront of my mind when I play, but my playing style is informed by what I have learned.

I certainly don't intend to convey the impression that the road map I have tried to carefully outline above is the only way to get to the land of Ecstasy. There are other approaches that work as well, maybe even better. I intend no criticism of them here. For me, I know how this one works, and that it can work well and consistently.

I share this information because I want Tops and bottoms to have better and more fulfilling scenes with each other. This makes a bigger pool of knowledgeable and experienced people out there for me to (hopefully) encounter at some later time. Seeds cast out into the wind. Perhaps some will come back to me one day.

Fear Is The Enemy

For the last 20 years or so, conventional wisdom in the SM scene has held that bottoms outnumbered Tops by a wide margin. Different people like to throw out different figures, but it is common to hear that there is one Top for every 10-15 bottoms. Various explanations have been offered to account for this numerical difference, but I have come not to believe it. What I do believe is that, historically, it has been much easier for bottoms to deal with their needs to submit (at least superficially) than it has been for Tops to deal much at all with their needs to dominate others.

In spite of the fact that men in American society get lots of support for being dominant, taking and using power, being a leader, making decisions, knowing what they want, and other traits usually associated with being a Top, most men sharply limit the ways in which they will allow their dominance and/or sadism to surface. The majority of them can do it only indirectly or symbolically, say perhaps when listening to the ecstatic conflicts that run through the music of Mahler or Vaughn Williams. Or maybe they get their dominant/sadistic rocks off vicariously by watching sporting events with heavy contact as in boxing, wrestling, or football; or perhaps when watching films with villains like Skeletor, Don Corleone, Lex Luthor, or powerful and destructive heros like Conan, Rambo, or the Terminator.

So why don't more guys come out more directly with their Top stuff, say, in an SM context? Why do they keep it hidden? For a while now, I have suspected that the reason more men don't let their dominance manifest itself in a more directly erotic way has to do with the fear and guilt they feel when they come face to face with the magnitude of their needs to be sadistic, their urges to control, and to dominate. It is as though

229

they sense the presence of some anarchic, lusty beast within themselves who could run wild and destroy everyone and everything in its path if released. So, many men keep the beasts within themselves safely caged except, perhaps, during private masturbations.

While most men may prefer to let their dominance and sadism out in largely symbolic ways, leathermen do it more directly during the SM scenes that we love. In some ways, SM scenes are where Tops test their abilities to let their inner beasts loose for long enough to gain lusty satisfaction, yet keep them restrained enough to prevent chaos and erotic anarchy from causing the true destruction that comes with unwanted consequences.

This delicate balancing act on the razor's edge between the urge to rape, pillage and destroy and the need for self-restraint is a battle that takes place behind the steely eyes of the sadist, the dominant. The tension created by this battle releases a flood of endorphin driven ecstatic pleasure that is unequaled. For me, and I suspect for many of us, this pleasure is one answer to the often asked question, "What do Tops get out of the scene, anyway?" As Thom Magister has pointed out, "He who would master another must first master himself."

At long last, there is some evidence that an increasing number of guys out there are becoming willing and able to come to terms with their own needs to dominate others and/or let their sadism out of its cage. This is probably because of the increased support for Tops that has become available in the last 10 years.

The wealth of technical information that has become available through publications, videos, workshops and demonstrations has helped Tops give real shape to their longings. At the same time, it has taught us how to be safer. These tools have given us the support and encouragement necessary to conquer our inner fears of our own dominance and sadism. More and more guys have begun to learn how to let the sadistic "monster" out of its cage for short periods, yet still keep it on a strong leash. This welcome development should produce a gradual equalization in the ratio of Tops to bottoms.

Having said all this, it is time to come to the point of this essay. For Tops to engage in this inner battle, we need and must have co-participation from brave and willing bottoms, and these, it turns out, are all too rare. It is not too hard to find bottoms who are willing to take a few steps with us as we make the journey, but most bottoms become paralyzed by their own fears long before we Tops get close to where we need to go. Bottoms who can go the distance with us are rare as hen's teeth.

Tops *need* such bottoms, for it is they who become the arena in which, and on which Tops test themselves. Bottoms are the necessary witnesses to, and participants in this drama. They watch us play with holy fire, and accompany us as each scene reconfirms us in a rite of passage. We re-affirm ourselves by mastering the inner impulses to destroy that remain from childhood. Only children and madmen destroy spontaneously for pleasure; true men create.

During SM scenes—the kinds of self-confrontational scenes I mentioned earlier—Tops edge ever closer to their internal "beasts," and take their bottoms along. Tops must draw near enough to the animal to collar him, then walk him in front of themselves through a cathartic portal, and beyond into transformation. But we can only go as close to that animal as bottoms will allow, for there must always be consent. Children take what they want for they have no interest in consent. These, though, are rites of passage for grownups.

"But you are asking us to jump into a Black Hole with you!" a famous slave protested recently in a discussion about this stuff. "Yes," I replied, "I am, and together we will come out on the other side of that Hole, The Cathartic Portal, having been profoundly changed by the passage." This idea instantly brings up two crucial issues for bottoms: First, how do I, as a bottom, know (trust?) that this particular Top can navigate the two of us successfully through what the slave called "The Black Hole," so we will come out safely on the other side? In effect, how do I know I will survive the experience, and not be

231

destroyed in there? (Remember: The black holes in the world of astrophysics are places where all matter is crushed together by heavy gravity and fused—places of death and rebirth.) Second, will I, as a bottom, be able to deal with (or even want) the changes that will happen to me as a result of the transformational passage?

I understand instantly what these questions mean. Remembering my years as a bottom, I recall the many times I asked myself what the SM scene would do to me if I continued my explorations in it. I asked myself if it would destroy me. I asked if I would like who I would be changed into; whether I would respect myself later; whether I would still be able to work and be productive; whether I would end up alone. Will I lose my old friends? Can I make new ones? I wondered whether I would still recognize the person that was essentially "Guy." All of these questions put me right up against my fears. The questions scared me. I somehow *knew* it was out there, and The Black Hole scared me greatly. I wanted guarantees that my passage into the Hole would not destroy me. In 1968, I stopped doing scenes for two years while I wrestled with these issues. And I remember the struggle well.

Finally, I was forced to accept that passage through the Cathartic Portal, the Black Hole, would indeed change me; that a part of me would die, and that I would be reborn in some way that was, finally, unpredictable. There were, I discovered, no guarantees of any kind whatsoever.

We must all come to terms with the fact that life itself changes us. Medical school changes the people who goes through it. Travel to the moon changes those who go there. Winning the lottery changes us. Losing a lover to disease changes us. Standing on a frontier, looking off into the distant unknown, looking towards the Black Hole, challenges us to risk change. And change is scary shit. The possibility of profound transformation is scarier still. But there it is. And every time we begin a scene, a part of us wonders if we will catch a glimpse of the Black Hole. That part wonders if we will take our next steps towards the thing. Wonders if this time we will step up to

232

the threshold itself, and peer into the swirling ethers of transformation, and perhaps surrender to them.

Clearly, the Black Hole experience—and the rites of passage that take us through it—these are the beacons toward which many of us travel in the SM scene. Some only sense them out there, somewhere in the darkness. Others can see them shining dimly, afar. For a few, they come fully into focus when we play. Fewer still enter.

I have already offered my view of the magic path Tops must take to confirm themselves, and of course, there is a corresponding path for bottoms. It lies parallel to the Top path, but is different. Along the bottom path, bottoms confront their essential vulnerability and triumph in survival. To really do this, and not just play at it, the bottom's vulnerability must be damn real—which it is when bottoms accompany Tops on their quest to collar the animals within themselves. This, I suspect, is the reason that bottoms are interested in testing their limits. It makes their vulnerability real, and it keeps their surrender meaningful. It amplifies that surrender until the surrender itself has enough power to change those who really can surrender.

And yes, real vulnerability is scary stuff. It must be so before it can do the job in a scene. The fear and intensity tells you that the vulnerability is authentic. It is upon this platform of vulnerability that Tops master their internal beasts. It is at this moment, this place which lies within the Black Hole, that Tops and bottoms fuse and become one. We go together, or else, we don't go at all.

After I was able to overcome the paralyzing fear that halted my bottom explorations for those two, dark years, my subsequent experiences in scenes confirmed to me that what I had feared would destroy me, instead had created and recreated me. They confirmed that the transformational passage caused me to feel more alive than ever before. My confidence grew. My self-esteem blossomed. I could love; I could sustain adventure and ecstasy. Bottoms who can truly surrender are the ones who learn to walk among the stars.

Well, the stage is now set. We have spent years making

technical, psychological, and emotional information available to Tops and bottoms alike. At endless workshops, seminars, and discussion groups our village elders have poured forth information at every opportunity: information to help Tops wrestle with their own frightening animals; and information to help bottoms wrestle with their own frightening vulnerabilities. For those who have mastered these techniques, the moment of truth is upon us. It comes down to this: can we find the courage within ourselves to deal with our fears (without drugs and alcohol, thank you) and to surrender to our respective quests, the ones completed, if ever, within the confines of the Black Hole?

We must. Otherwise, we all risk being reduced to male impersonators or, at best, sport fuckers. And *no*, this is not just macho posturing. After all, the purpose of rites of passage is to confirm something to those who are performing the rite. To undertake the rite without making the passage simply reduces us to being ritualists or liturgists—empty and meaningless—the jewel box without the jewel. If we are ultimately going to be unwilling or unable to one day actually undertake the passage itself, then why would we step into the ritual chamber in the first place? To only do SM "just for fun" is to waste the trip. To visit The Vatican just to look at the art there misses the main point of the place.

I, like Gayle Rubin and many others, hate perfunctory SM: attach shackle "A" to wrist "B"; then do this and say that. The "paint-by-number" experience—formula SM—does not produce masterpieces for anyone. Perfunctory SM, or something like it, may be a necessary step toward achieving the skills required to undertake transforming experiences, but to get stuck there reduces us to being mere technicians. It does not produce artists, nor does it give us the navigation skills that can take us successfully toward and through the Cathartic Portal. Playing all the musical notes correctly as written in a piece of music does not necessarily produce music.

For me, this scene is ultimately all about confrontation with Self. Bottoms confront one facet of the Self; Tops confront a

234

different facet. And, we all have both facets, all of us are potential switches—both Top and bottom, Sadist and masochist, Master and slave. Fear of these confrontations can stop both Tops and bottoms long before they get anywhere near the threshold of The Black Hole experience. For Tops, some fear is necessary to prevent us from moving too far and too fast during a scene. For bottoms, some fear is necessary to prevent them from connecting with crazy or incompetent Tops. But the fear that leads to paralysis—to the lack of will to move toward the Black Hole experience—*this* fear is our enemy for it can prevent us from taking the transformational journey.

This fear is my enemy. I think it is our enemy. I challenge you to master yours, and step through the temple doors into the ritual chamber to be changed there. Changed into yourSelf.

"...for many are called, but few are chosen."—From the Parable of the Wedding Feast

Mr. Baldwin wishes to give special thanks to J.K., R.B. and j.b. #3 for comments and feedback on this piece.

In My Father's House,
There Are Many Mansions

When I was in college, I recall hearing something said by a guru named Baba Ram Dass. It went something like this: "Many paths lead to the pyramid's summit, but which ever one you choose, the view from the top is always the same."

It has always been relatively easy to talk about the technical parts of the SM/leather scene—how to handle a whip or do an electrical scene—probably because these things aren't very personal. So, we learn, "Attach shackle (A) to wrist (B)...," and so on. While this kind of information is certainly important, there are other aspects of the leather/SM experience that we have very carefully avoided mentioning for too long.

One man in Texas said to me, "My buddies would laugh at me if I told them what happens in my mind sometimes when I play." So, he doesn't tell, and they don't laugh. As you may have guessed, he was referring to the spiritual—transcendental? mystical?—experiences he has when he plays.

This guy is not alone. Many feel that it is not hot, or not butch to admit to such thoughts. Leather dykes have been talking openly about the spiritual angles of the leather/SM scene for a long time, but most men are still shy about bringing them up.

It may come as a surprise to some of you, but the leather/SM lifestyle does bring up spiritual and religious issues for lots of guys in the scene. A man in New York with a Pentecostal background is concerned about his salvation; another wants information about his out-of-body experiences when in bondage. Fears about demonic possession dominate a guy who takes me aside to chat about it in Seattle. A Catholic in Dallas asks me about becoming a monk so that, maybe, he can whip himself without risking sin. A guy from Denver writes to ask about a possible relationship between meditation and submission. Another asks if he is confusing endorphins with spiritual ecstasy.

These things come up in the therapy room. And, it seems to me, the people who have the most trouble dealing with their SM/leather interests are those who grew up believing that it is dangerous to make up one's own mind about God (and, often, about one's own self as well).

When churches and churchmen are the final authority about God, leather/SM urges present a real conflict. I have run into more than one bottom with a fundamentalist upbringing who suspected that Tops might be Satan incarnate. Such people fear for their souls every time they play.

"Is this stuff going to send me straight to Hell?" "Am I doing spiritual damage to myself when I do sadistic things to someone or want them done to me?" "Maybe even the fantasies about leather/SM are dangerous and could hurt my chances for eternal life."

Questions like these might seem silly if you have decided that God is a man-made myth or that He does not really give a damn how you live your life. But if you are someone for whom God is Fact, and you believe that He has clear laws about the Right and Wrong of how to behave, then what you do with a whip could matter. Should it?

Each of us, of course, must make peace with himself about God and go on with life. The important thing here is that we not be afraid to ask ourselves honest questions in the search for a truth we can live with confidently. We can do this, and we must. Changes in the attitudes we encounter in the leather scene today are making this easier to do.

New Age consciousness is moving through the leather scene, slowly changing the way that leatherfolks relate to each other both in and out of the playroom. New Age morality and spirituality is "allowing," tolerant and experimental.

Younger leathermen who were investigating New Age

238

attitudes before they got into leather expect their leatherlife to resonate with new age ideals. Sometimes, New Agers have had a rough time fitting leather/SM stuff into their morality partly because the Old Guard Leathermen don't tolerate much diversity.

When the spiritual aspects of SM/leather/fetish sexualities are paid attention to, they can add to who we are as people by increasing intimacy. As I have often said, sexualities that keep us apart only diminish us as people.

It is not outrageous to suggest the possibility that those of us who pursue ecstatic spiritual or mystical experience through SM/leather/fetish actions may be the early forerunners of a new spiritual tradition. Anybody want to start a Church? After all, this is supposed to be the country that, first and foremost, protects religious freedom. It could be fun to put that principal to the test. It could also be a pain in the ass.

In any case, I hope that my public comments, including this book, will stimulate your thinking about these issues, and, perhaps more importantly, stimulate conversation with your kinky buddies. Those of us who have or seek these experiences need to come out of our closets about this part of the SM/leather/fetish scene. We need to read and write about it more. After all, we must be free to speak our minds about anything. Right?

ABOUT THE AUTHOR

Guy Baldwin, M.S., is a psychotherapist in private practice in Los Angeles where he works primarily with those on the erotic frontiers. In demand as a guest speaker and teacher, he has traveled the U.S. and Canada to offer a wide array of workshops and seminars to audiences of leather folks. He has been a featured presenter at the annual convention of the National Leather Association for the last five years.

Mr. Baldwin's television appearances include interviews on *A.M. Philadelphia*, on *The Gay Cable Network* in New York City, San Francisco, and Portland, Oregon; other interviews include *CBS Talk Radio, Florida*, and various gay and lesbian newspapers. He is perhaps best known for his numerous articles about leather/SM-related issues which appeared primarily in *Drummer* magazine between 1987 and 1992. Other articles were published in *Manifest Reader, Frontiers, The Leather Journal* and *Checkmate*. Most are collected in this volume. His essay, *A Second Coming Out* appeared in *Leatherfolk*, a collection of essays edited for Alyson Publications (1991) by Mark Thompson. Baldwin has also written *The Leather Contest Handbook: A Handbook for Promoters, Contestants, Judges and Titleholders*.

In 1989-90, he served as the eleventh International Mr. Leather and the second Mr. National Leather Association.

To receive a catalog and mail order information write to:

Daedalus Publishing Company
2140 Hyperion Ave.
Los Angeles, CA 90027

Or send e-mail to:

Info@daedaluspublishing.com

Or send fax to:

323-913-5976

Or visit our web site at:

http://www.daedaluspublishing.com

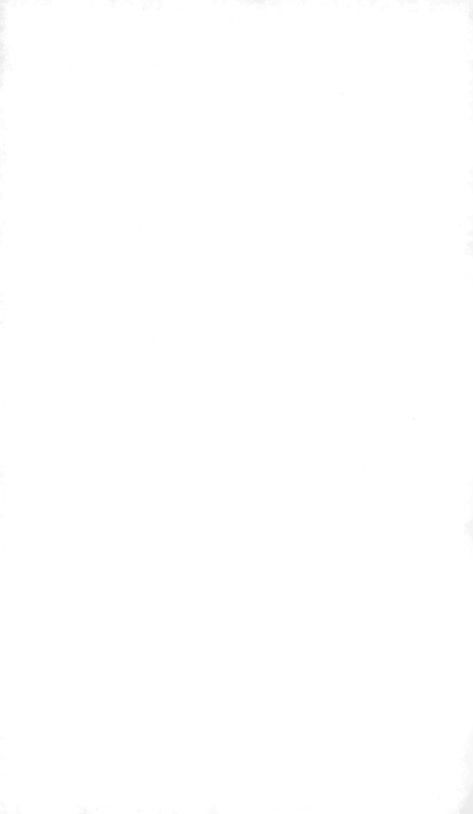